Building Bridges

The future of GP education – developing partnerships with the service

Building Bridges

The future of GP education – developing partnerships with the service

Edited by Steve Gillam, John Eversley,
Janet Snell & Paul Wallace

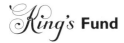

Published by
King's Fund Publishing
11–13 Cavendish Square
London W1M 0AN

First published 1999

ISBN 1 85717 231 0

A CIP catalogue record for this book is available from the British Library

Available from:
King's Fund Bookshop
11–13 Cavendish Square
London
W1M 0AN

Tel: 0171 307 2591
Fax: 0171 307 2801

Printed and bound in Great Britain

Cover illustration: Minuche Mazumdar Farrar

Contents

Contributors

Maggie Aiken, Postgraduate Education Manager, Queen Mary and Westfield College

Tom Bolger, Assistant General Secretary, Royal College of Nursing

Isobel Bowler, Nottingham University LIZ GP Incentives Evaluation Team

Robert Boyd, Principal, St George's Hospitals Medical School, London

Charles Easmon, Director of Education and Training, NHSE, London Regional Office

John Eversley, Senior Research Fellow, Queen Mary and Westfield College, London

Jon Fuller, Senior Lecturer, Imperial College School of Medicine

Madeleine Gantley, Senior Lecturer, Dept of General Practice & Primary Care, Queen Mary & Westfield College

Steve Gillam, Director, Primary Care Programme, King's Fund

Judy Gilley, Joint Deputy Chairman, General Practitioner Committee (GPC)

Trisha Greenhalgh, Senior Lecturer, Royal Free and University College Schools of Medicine, London

Iona Heath, north London GP

Alison Hill, Senior Lecturer, Queen Mary and Westfield College

Alex Jamieson, Associate Dean, Thames Postgraduate Medical and Dental Education

Diana Kelly, Lecturer in Medical Education, King's College School of Medicine and Dentistry

Anne Kilcoyne, Research Co-ordinator, Department of General Practice, Imperial College School of Medicine, London

Philip Leech, Principal Medical Officer, Department of Health

Roger Murphy, Nottingham University LIZ GP Incentives Evaluation Team

Geoffrey Norris, Associate Dean, Thames Post-graduate Medical and Dental Education

Roland Petchey, Nottingham University LIZ GP Incentives Evaluation Team

Patrick Pietroni, Postgraduate Dean of General Practice, North Thames

Tony Rennison, IT Educationalist, Queen Mary and Westfield College

Jo Tissier, Research Assistant, Department of General Practice and Primary Care, Queen Mary and Westfield College

Paul Wallace, Professor, Royal Free and University College Schools of Medicine

Susan Williams, Joint Chief Executive, Barking & Havering Health Authority

Preface

General practice is in a phase of rapid development. In the course of the last ten years, it has moved quite dramatically to occupy a centre-stage position in the NHS. On the one hand, GPs find themselves responsible with other primary care colleagues for a growing range of health care provision of increasing complexity and sophistication. On the other, they have been asked to take a crucial role in commissioning health care services, first through fundholding and now through the establishment of primary care groups. And if all this were not enough for a profession made up largely of independent contractors to the NHS, general practice is increasingly called upon to provide a growing range of educational opportunities at both the undergraduate and postgraduate level and to take a greater role in research.

In common with other medical specialties, general practice is also facing a massive growth in the volume and complexity of the knowledge base which practitioners need to have in order to ensure that the care which they offer their patients is of the highest quality. In the new information era, pressure comes not only from health care managers demanding greater levels of professional accountability in the form of clinical governance, but also from patients with increasing access to a wide range of sources of information about their health problems. In order to keep abreast of these massive changes there is an imperative as never before for members of the primary health care team to undertake effective programmes of continuing medical education and professional development.

General practice has responded in different ways to these issues. While many GPs have welcomed the changes, taking the initiative in developing their practices, undertaking new responsibilities and forming new alliances, morale in the profession as a whole has been steadily falling and there have been serious problems both with retention of established GP principals and with recruitment to the specialty. These problems are not confined to GPs, but extend to the full range of primary care professionals. In London the situation has been particularly severe, and concerns about the poor state of general practice in the capital prompted a number of major governmental initiatives.

One of these, the London Initiative Zone Educational Incentives (LIZEI) programme, was designed specifically to address this problem by stimulating the provision of funded opportunities for GPs to undertake educational activities. Although a number of specific objectives for the scheme were announced at its launch, the general aim was to ensure the involvement of as many as possible of the GPs practising within the London Initiative Zone (LIZ) area. The realisation of the programme depended crucially on the formation of a novel set of alliances between individual GPs, local medical committees, educational groupings in both the university and postgraduate sectors and health care managers. Despite a good deal of initial scepticism and an almost impossibly tight time schedule, the three-year LIZEI programme succeeded remarkably in involving more than three-quarters of the eligible GPs.

The range of educational activities undertaken was enormous (see Chapter 3), but one constant factor emerged as crucial for the programme's success, namely an alliance centred on the education–service partnership. Support for this became increasingly evident as the programme progressed and led to the establishment of the London Education Service Partnership (LESP), an alliance of most of the organisations involved with LIZEI, whose task was to examine how to build on the lessons learned from the programme about linking education and service in general practice, not only within London but across the UK as a whole (see Appendix).

LESP convened a one-day symposium at the King's Fund in February 1998, the aim of which was to bring together key players from general practice, the NHS and academia to examine in some detail the main issues relating to the development of the education–service partnership in general practice. The symposium generated a remarkable response from the one hundred or so participants and there was a powerful sense of the relevance and importance of this issue for the development of general practice now and in the future. One of the clearest messages to emerge from the meeting was the need both for the development of national provision to facilitate and stimulate the education–service partnership in general practice and for the establishment of local groups to undertake the necessary practical steps.

This book draws heavily but not exclusively on the symposium. New material has been commissioned. The contributions read in sequence but can also stand alone. The book provides a record of past achievement; indeed it begins with a historical review of GP education. But it should also act as a stimulus for the continuing development of an alliance between education and service in general practice. This should have benefits for patients, GPs and other primary health care professionals, and for those with responsibility for management within the NHS.

Steve Gillam, John Eversley, Janet Snell and Paul Wallace

Acknowledgements
We are grateful to Stuart Drage, Neil Jackson and other members of the LESP Steering Group. To Nigel Oswald for comments on previous drafts.

Abbreviations

BMA	British Medical Association
CeMENT	Community-based Medical Education in North Thames programme
CHI	Commission for Health Improvement
CME	Continuing medical education
CMO	Chief Medical Officer
CPD	Continuing professional development
FHSA	Family health services authority
GMC	General Medical Council
GMSC	General Medical Services Committee (now GPC)
GP	General practitioner
HA	Health authority
JCPTGP	Joint Committee on Postgraduate Training for General Practice
LIZ	London Initiative Zone
LIZEI	London Initiative Zone Educational Incentives programme
MAAG	Medical audit advisory group
MADEL	Medical and dental education levy
MRCGP	Member of the Royal College of General Practitioners
NICE	National Institute of Clinical Excellence
NMET	Non-medical education and training
PCG	Primary care group
PDP	Personal development plan
PEP	Personal education plan
PGEA	Postgraduate education accreditation
PGMDE	Postgraduate medical and dental education
PREP	Post-registration education and practice
REDG	Regional educational development group
SIFT	Service increments for teaching

Chapter 1

Many rivers to cross: medical education and general practice

John Eversley

KEY POINTS

- The nature of preparation for general practice and the professional development of general practitioners (GPs) depends on what general practice and primary care are perceived to be about. There is not a consensus on this and therefore preparation and development need to be pluralist in their approaches

- Medical education has changed little over the last hundred years

- In the development of GPs as in many other professions and occupations, a distinction is often made between 'education' and 'training'. Here, it is argued that this distinction is unsustainable in theory and undesirable in practice and so the terms are used interchangeably. It is suggested that the model of 'experiential learning' is preferable to 'education plus training'

- The development and accreditation of GPs have been dominated by training in, and for, hospital medicine, although this is changing

- The number of institutions involved in medical education, and the planning and delivery of services, contributes to its complexity and resistance to change

- Learning and professional development for general practice will have to change radically in the face of new challenges within the NHS and higher education

General practice and primary care: the implications for education

Vuori (1996) has suggested that primary care is:

- a level of care
- a set of activities
- a strategy for organising health services
- a philosophy for a health care system.

The implications of this are explored below but it is important to highlight that primary care has changed with time and place. When Lord Dawson coined the phrase 'primary care' in 1920, he had his experience as an officer in World War I in mind. He saw primary care as first aid in the trenches, backed up by field stations and hospitals behind the lines (Honigsbaum 1979). When the World Health Organization talks about primary care globally, it includes clean water and adequate nutrition. Historically and globally, primary care has not been equated with general medical practice. However, in the UK context in the 1990s, a 'primary care-led NHS' with primary care groups appears to mean a general-practitioner-led system. Following Vuori, we can analyse the implications for education and training of different perspectives on primary care.

Primary care as a level of care

Primary care is the first level of formal care in contrast to self-care, secondary or tertiary care. If general practice is thought of as a level of care, then an essential skill of practitioners will be to know when to intervene or refer onwards. GPs need to know what others in the health care system are capable of without necessarily being able to do the task themselves. They do not necessarily need to know how hospital doctors perform particular procedures but they may need to know how to access meals on wheels or housing adaptations. Prospective GPs are unlikely to learn this from hospital doctors but might learn it from practising GPs, social workers, occupational therapists or housing officers.

Primary care as a strategy

Perspectives on primary care are suffused with military analogies. According to the Oxford English Dictionary, the term 'strategy' is derived from ancient Greek warfare: the art or plan of the commander in chief for winning a war, as opposed to 'tactics' for winning a battle. The term is often used interchangeably with 'models' or 'philosophies'. Discussion of health care strategies can take us back to first principles about the relationships between mind, body and the environment (Engel 1997). Two slightly different medical models will be addressed here. George Engel's thinking has been influential internationally and he has specifically considered the implications of different models for medical education. Peter Toon (1994) is a London GP who was employed by the NHS Executive (North Thames) to co-ordinate the LIZEI programme.

Engel contrasts the biomedical model with a biopsychosocial model. The biomedical model explains disease in terms of measurable biological variables. He argues that this is the dominant medical model both within the medical profession and within western societies. The biopsychosocial model which Engel proposes takes into account:

● the patient's experience of the disease ('illness')
● the impact of mental states on physical well-being and on response to treatment
● the importance of living conditions on disease and illness
● psychological and social factors in determining whether a patient views themselves, or is viewed as, sick
● the relationship between the doctor and patient.

Toon identifies three broad approaches influencing general practice:

● a biomedical model (substantially the same as Engel's)
● a humanist model (for example, the work of Balint)
● a public health model (for example, the work of Julian Tudor Hart).

Essentially Engel's model draws the humanist and public health models together. Observation of many London GPs suggests that they do likewise.

The biomedical doctor needs to be taught primarily how to diagnose, treat and cure biological abnormality. Learning about technological wizardry and absorbing biological facts are likely to be central to medical education. For the biopsychosocial or humanist doctor, developing interpersonal skills and an ability to draw out and use patients' understanding of their condition will be critical. A doctor taking the public health perspective needs to learn about the economic and social causes and consequences of morbidity and well-being and how doctors can influence these.

In reality, these models are not mutually exclusive. The debate within medical education is more about how much of each doctor needs to know. In the twentieth century medical education has been dominated by the biomedical model at the expense of the humanist or public health approaches.

Primary care as a philosophy

General practice in the UK is a free, universal, voluntary, demand-led system that acts as a gatekeeper to most of secondary and tertiary care. There are various qualifications to this in practice but this both describes the aim of the system and the substance of what actually occurs.

> 'The family doctor or community nurse is often the first port of call for patients when they need health advice or treatment. Primary care professionals are also the way into the NHS for most patients. They understand patients' needs and they deliver most local services. That is why they will be in the driving seat in shaping local health services in the future.' (DoH 1997)

The above statement mixes description with inference and prescription and it has major implications for medical education. Although practitioners are the point of entry to health care, this does not automatically mean that practitioners understand patients' needs. Training, information and resources to help assess needs are required. Shaping local services requires specific skills and knowledge and even tests of competence. It is by no means obvious that, because GPs and nurses are in the 'front line' (a military analogy again), they should lead. It turns centuries of feudalism, capitalism, military organisation and public services management on its head to argue that the people in the front line should direct the whole enterprise. If family doctors and community nurses are to play these roles, how are they to learn them? The responsibilities imply understanding people and financial management on a vastly different scale from that of a general practice.

Primary care as a set of activities

Bosanquet (1996) divides GP work into four categories:

- demand-led consultations
- disease management
- identifying risk factors for disease and screening
- referral to/organising secondary care.

General medical services have for the last 120 years at least been defined as 'what an average GP does'. But the role changes. Both the 1990 contract and the GMSC work (GMSC 1996) on defining core and non-core services have widened the specification of what a GP should do. Nevertheless, GPs often express great hostility to any prescription of what they must or must not do. Clearly, what the activities of general practice are or what they should be has profound implications for education and training.

Education and training: an unsustainable distinction

Writers on medical education are generally confident that there is a difference:

> 'Training, often on the apprenticeship model, is characterised by a sequence of instruction followed by practice under supervision with feedback on performance and assessment of competence and prepares the doctor to respond competently to familiar patterns and situations, often with little critical thinking.
>
> 'Education on the other hand is a broader concept and involves specific teaching and learning strategies, which in contrast to training encourages critical thinking and the ability to solve unfamiliar problems by the application of the knowledge gained from such teaching and learning'. (Lister 1993)

The training/education distinction goes to the heart of the question of why a partnership might be needed between 'education' and 'service'. It is a debate that extends far beyond medicine. But the distinction does not bear close scrutiny and indeed, in practice, the terms are often used interchangeably.

The training/education distinction also masks the important function of education or training in initiating or socialising individuals so that they conform to the norms of an occupation. This can be presented either as a high-minded requirement to achieve the ethical standards of a profession or as a more mundane way of ensuring that members' first loyalty is to 'the club'. It may also be both.

The traditional apprenticeship model (codified by the Statute of Artificers of 1563) included observation, assisting the craftsman, 'set pieces', journeyman status and becoming a craftsman (Perry 1976). At the heart of the distinction is that 'gentlemen are educated and tradesmen are trained' (Downie and Charlton 1992). Apprenticeship, general practice and pursuit of a trade have been associated. On the other hand, physicians have been 'educated'. The shift during the first half of the nineteenth century from an apprenticeship model to a medical school model may have had precisely the intention of shifting the social status of doctors from tradesmen to gentlemen by excluding poorer people from training.

The idea that education is for the sake of learning and training is for employment creates an artificial distinction. Education for the mass of the population has always been thought relevant to employment. The Society for the Diffusion of Useful Knowledge was launched in the nineteenth century and recently we have seen the New Vocationalism of the 1980s – though there have been challenges to this view too (CCCS 1981).

Regulation of training has always been closely related to the control of entry to occupations in order to regulate wages or to maintain standards. However, education has also reflected labour market pressures.

Training has also been linked to an 'incentive' model, by which it is assumed that individuals and employers both benefit from training but that both need sticks and carrots to encourage them. The same has been true for education (Perry 1976, Simon 1974). The need for incentives for employers is based on the assumption that a trainee is less productive and produces lower-quality work than a qualified person. Furthermore, if there were not incentives to train, employers would simply 'pay and poach', i.e. pay a premium to get a skilled workforce. Typically, in the world outside medicine, the most junior entrants are paid least and subsidised least. Most of their training is 'on the job' but involves doing rather than training by doing. Logic might dictate that the most junior staff should be subsidised more and receive more off-the-job training.

Neither the 'education' nor the 'training' paradigms are separable from questions about what knowledge is, what skills are, why and how people learn, who learns and what learning is for. In the wider world of adult education 'experiential' learning has been recognised as increasingly important.

Apprenticeship is based on the importance of passing on the teacher's experience to the learner, who adds to their learning by their experience. Most of the major educational traditions incorporate the learner's life experience in some way (Saddington, 1992). For instance, in the Socratic tradition the learner has to have a basic knowledge and understanding in order to have a dialogue with the teacher who constructs and delivers wisdom. In the Progressive tradition, educationalists such as Dewey see the learner as teacher but nonetheless needing to learn how to learn. Even in the Behaviourist or technological tradition of those like Lewin and Skinner, the learner's life experiences determine the entry point for the learning process. Unless we reduce 'experiential' to anything which takes account of experience, we need to be more specific about what it means and why it might be useful in the formation of health professionals.

Experiential learning

The concept of experiential learning, as used in adult education, embraces:

- assessing and accrediting life and work experience as a route to professional recognition
- changing the way students learn within formal education
- education to promote social change
- promoting personal growth and development (Weil and McGill 1989).

With the development of knowledge, skills and changes in attitudes, drawn out from the experience of the learners in a planned way, experiential learning represents a synthesis of what the separate worlds of education and training may be about.

Science versus craft

'Better to send a man to Oxford to be instructed in shoemaking than to learn how to practise medicine.' Thomas Sydenham (see Weatherall 1993)

While the training/education distinction and the relevance of experiential learning and theory have been debated outside medicine, within the profession different terms are used. A contrast has been made between the 'science' versus the 'craft' (the specialty committees of the BMA are still called craft committees) or 'humanitarian' approaches. This debate has been going on for a long time.

In the seventeenth century, Thomas Sydenham argued for the primacy of observation and experiment over theory. He felt that the curriculum of his time involved too much talking and not enough healing (Whitehouse, Roland and Campion 1997). The Flexner report before the first world war argued for a basic science training as a foundation for clinical training and the separation of pre-clinical and clinical training or theory and practice (Schön 1991). In the 1920s and 1930s Henry Brackenbury, a North London GP, argued for a social model of medicine and an education based on experience (see Box below). On the other hand, Lord Dawson, the physician at the London Hospital who coined the term 'primary care' in the UK, argued for more science and a narrower clinical training (Honigsbaum 1979).

A GP's VIEW IN 1935

Just in case we should run away with the idea that any of the debates about medical education in the late 1990s are anything new, the writings of Henry Brackenbury should remind us that we have been here before. Brackenbury was a GP in Hornsey, North London, chairman of the BMA in 1930s as well as a Labour politician and influential in debates about the founding of the NHS. He argued against a narrow focus of medical education on biology. Medicine was immensely indebted to many sciences but dependent on none. He was excited by the discoveries around immunisation, genetics and what he called the 'new psychology' but also very much interested in the whole person and people's economic and social conditions. He argued that for a surprisingly long period not very much attention seemed to have been paid to anything wider than the family environment and that the volume of preventive work being done by GPs was not generally appreciated. Health has to be preserved as well as restored – he used the term 'perfective health'. Medical schools ought to pay much more attention to teaching doctors how to learn what was going on in the patient's mind. 'It would be a good thing,' he argued, 'if the medical student, as part of his course, had to share an appropriate portion of a nurse's training, not only that he might be the more fully equipped to direct, supervise and appraise, but that he might have greater knowledge of the ways of adding to the patient's comfort.'

He suggested that: 'It would not be without compensating advantage if every doctor, early in his active career, were to experience at least one serious illness'. He also highlighted one of the enduring issues of continuing medical education: 'There are many opportunities for postgraduate training but there are many doctors who, owing of their locality or the circumstances of their practice, find immense difficulty in availing themselves'.

Undergraduate medical education in the UK has been anything but 'experiential', as defined above. It has, however, included substantial experience: in the eighteenth, nineteenth (and arguably the twentieth) centuries the dominant model in medicine was: 'See one, do one, teach one' (Lowry 1993). Two of the characteristics of a narrow approach to vocational preparation, namely the 'factual overload' and the passive acquisition of knowledge, have been criticised by the GMC's education committee for decades (Lister 1993). Experiential learning in medicine today is more likely to be called 'problem-based learning' or 'self-directed learning' and to have entered the lives of students mainly after they have graduated. However, the introduction of objective structured clinical examinations (OSCEs) as the final test for undergraduates is changing this.

Downie and Charlton suggest that, to an outsider, medical education looks like a process of 'indoctrination or professionalisation'; to a social scientist, it is a process of establishing standards of conformity, and that it is also a 'progressive desensitisation to the patients' point of view' (Downie and Charlton 1992). Building *esprit de corps* and shutting out other professions and users seem to be a characteristic of professional training, but there have also been movements to change this (Schön 1991).

Regulation of entry and control of training have been closely linked in medicine. Before the creation of the NHS, the profession and the state debated how many doctors were needed and how to avoid 'over-doctoring' – specifically in order not to undermine the incomes of existing ones. Control over who could train and over numbers trained was used to ensure that there were not too many doctors. In the 1980s, the debate about motivation to learn was reflected in the arguments about whether a 'good practice allowance' was appropriate to general practice and whether it should be part of the remuneration package for GPs. The debate about incentives for employers is expressed as 'the core problem of reconciling educational requirements with service needs.' The debate about productivity and who pays is reflected partly in the service increment for teaching (SIFT) arrangements but also in the fact that the service commitments of junior hospital doctors have generally taken priority over their requirements for education and training (Lister 1993).

The stages of medical education

From the middle of the eighteenth century to the middle of the twentieth century, the aim of medical education was to produce a 'safe general practitioner ready on the day of qualification'. 'General practitioner' meant something wider than what would be understood by the same term today. Until 1978, the qualifying exam for doctors was in medicine, surgery and midwifery.

Various pressures have increased the amount of training GPs require:

- The existing pattern of training is not appropriate, for various reasons. Extra training has been added before and after qualification and throughout the later careers of GPs. The alternatives have not found much favour, for example: removing elements; changing the nature of training (less 'facts', more knowing where and how to find out, for example) or redefining roles so that different types of doctors do not all have the same basic training

- Changes in technology (including pharmaceutical advances) and wider shifts in the pattern of illness and care have added to the range of activities that can be carried out in general practice

- A growing view that not all training should be at the beginning of careers. Between the two world wars, a series of government and professional committees (Athlone and Cohen, for example) chipped away at the notion of training only until doctors were first qualified. The Royal Commission on Medical Education (Todd) did the same thing in 1968

- Economic and social pressures have also worked to extend the period of training. This includes the advantages of trainees as 'cheap labour'; public pressure to raise standards and a concern to raise the professional status of GPs by making an excess of demand over supply a mark of desirability. This has reflected the need to recruit and retain more doctors in general and more GPs in particular.

The resulting arrangements therefore embrace:

- undergraduate education
- vocational training
- continuing medical education.

All of these are underpinned by legislation and regulation. In addition, there are a host of other opportunities and resources for learning.

Undergraduate education

The thrust behind undergraduate education throughout most of the twentieth century has been to bring in a clinical 'science' curriculum. This was the 'Flexner' model first proposed in the USA, which spread through medical education in both the industrialised world and in those developing countries where medical education was influenced by colonial powers. As Hart (1988) says of the Flexner doctors:

> '*The new doctors needed no understanding of the anatomy or physiology of society, nor the social history of medicine [or people] for these may divert them from the acquisition of the apparently limitless facts of medical science, and were in any case useless.*'

An education foundation was added to an already-established apprenticeship model. Paradoxically, it built on the liberal arts tradition of educating the physicians.

Selection methods used

Walton (1977) asserted that the selection methods of students had more of an impact on output than teaching methods. But McManus (1989) found that learning styles are better predictors of university performance than A level results, which are given great weight in most selection processes. In 1998, this debate is still live with a shift away from reliance on A level results being demanded by the GMC.

Medical teachers

Medical teachers can be divided into three groups:

- a tiny minority who are trained in educational theory and methods and are often not medically qualified themselves
- staff holding official 'teaching' appointments but without formal teacher training
- NHS doctors who teach.

More medical schools are nowadays offering their staff training in educational methods or even requiring them to undertake this. However the teaching staff of medical schools are still overwhelmingly medical with the implication that the best people to teach doctors are other doctors. This does not always happen in other professions.

Attitudes to general practice

The medical schools actively resisted the re-introduction of the GP-based experiential teaching as 'educationally harmful' (Ellis 1979) when it was proposed by the GMC at the turn of the century.

Richards (1993) described the purpose of educating students outside hospital as:

> 'Not to train medical students to become general practitioners (although half the students will eventually go into general practice) but to show in surgeries and patients' own homes a different spectrum of disease, an approach appropriate to handling patients with minor everyday illnesses, and the different pattern of working conditions outside hospital. Insight, not instruction, is the keynote, a counterbalance to the rarefied atmosphere of hospital, an awareness essential for those concerned with partnership of care between hospital and general practice.' (Richards 1993)

The implications seem clear: general practice is pictured as being about minor illness; education is located in general practice so that students understand what is done there, not so that they learn how to do it.

Even McCormick (1992), a professor of general practice, said: 'There is no place for attempting to teach general practice to undergraduates'. Nevertheless, general practice has slowly carved a place in undergraduate education. In 1962, 17 out of 23 UK medical schools had voluntary GP attachments and three had compulsory attachments. By 1987 all schools had formal attachments in general practice (Fraser 1987). The move to base medical education in the community has steadily gathered momentum (Oswald 1989).

In 1963 the first UK professor of general practice was appointed in Edinburgh. In 1968 the Royal Commission on Medical Education, influenced by the Royal College of General Practitioners, 'rehabilitated' general practice. The College built on this and 'introduced educational objectives instead of the apprenticeship training pattern' (Walton 1997). (Note the implication that education is superior to training). Departments of General Practice became much more widespread in the 1970s. However it was not until the 1990s that professors in general practice were appointed in Oxford and Cambridge and even now there are a number of Departments of General Practice which are combined with other areas of medicine.

Vocational training

The first trainee scheme for GPs was launched by the Government in 1946. It provided for a one-year 'apprenticeship' as an assistant in general practice. The scheme lasted until 1966.

From the mid-1960s onwards, culminating in the Royal Commission on Medical Education (The Todd Report) in 1968, a series of reports recommended post-qualification training for general practice. The Todd Report recommended five years' training for general practice.

Although it was finally recommended that GPs should have three years' vocational training, it did not become compulsory for new principals until 1982. There are still many practising GPs who are not vocationally trained because they came into practice before 1982.

The first Vocational Training Scheme course organisers were appointed in 1972. Training of GP trainers and course organisers began in the early 1970s – before training for many university and hospital trainers became common. Even now, two out of three years of training for general practice are in a hospital setting. Although it is in specialties relevant to general practice, many doctors in training and many of their trainers are sceptical about its value as preparation for the role.

Attention to the methods used in vocational training was given at an early stage. The Joint Committee on Postgraduate Training for General Practice (see below) was responsible for issuing certificates of 'satisfactory completion' of vocational training. But right up to 1998, satisfactory completion could be on the basis of attendance or statements from trainers and consultants. In 1998 summative assessment (i.e. an assessment of the standard achieved at the end of training) became compulsory. The RCGP has put considerable effort into promoting the examination for the MRCGP but this has not been a compulsory exam and most GPs do not have the qualification. Writing in the early 1990s, Lister (1993) could find no evidence that vocational training makes better doctors. However a more recent review has found that there is generally a positive effect (Hindmarsh *et al.* 1998).

GPs have had a formalised gate-keeping role since the creation of the NHS. Since 1991, increasing numbers of GPs have been given responsibilities for commissioning secondary care and community services. However, training for these roles has been left to local discretion and attention to curriculum design, content and method has often been scant. As primary care groups take shape, it has so far been left to local initiative to decide what adjustments will be made to both vocational training and continuing professional development.

Continuing professional development

Continuing education for GPs first received direct state funding when Section 63 of the Health Services and Public Health Act 1968 was implemented. From 1968 to 1977 and then again from 1990, attendance at approved activities was a condition for payments to GPs – first as seniority allowances, later as postgraduate education allowances (PGEA).

There is only limited evidence that doctors who have had what became known as Continuing Medical Education (CME) are any more competent than those who have not (Lister 1993). Continuing medical education has often consisted of lectures by consultants after lunches paid for by pharmaceutical companies attended by more or less soporific GPs. Fortunately, there has been a shift towards self-directed and practice-based learning.

More GPs are becoming involved in teaching and research. This may be an important stimulus to continuing professional development. Accreditation as trainers and the development of research frequently involve peer scrutiny and heightened self-awareness.

The institutional base of medical education

The number and nature of different institutions involved in medical education contribute to its complexity. It is therefore important to understand how they came to be involved and something of their role. The arrangements that have evolved represent a division of education for general practice into largely independent 'countries' which, if they are not actually at war with each other, pursue their national interests. These do not always promote preparation for practice. The development of each of the institutions is considered in turn.

The General Medical Council

The GMC was established by the Medical Act 1858. A principal aim in establishing it was to outlaw quackery and alternative medicine. 'Quackery' was a term derived from the German term for 'mercury' (*Quacksilber*), which was used for treating syphilis at the time. Though this might have been a preoccupation of male legislators in the mid-nineteenth century – and later legislation specifically outlawed unqualified practitioners treating venereal disease – the term had come to mean medical practice by the unqualified. One of the Act's most far-reaching measures was that it instituted examinations as the route to qualification (Downie and Charlton 1992).

Crucially from the point of view of general practice, the constitution of the GMC was at first heavily weighted towards the universities and the existing corporations (mainly the royal colleges) and the influence of GPs was limited. Although this situation has evolved over the last 140 years, hospital medicine still has a disproportionate weight within the GMC. At the same time, the GMC's attempts to move medical education away from the hospital setting have met with limited success.

The royal colleges and higher training committees

The power of the royal colleges goes back to the medieval guild system in which examinations were a way of controlling entry. When the surgeons, physicians and apothecaries each founded their colleges, they were specifically modelled on medieval guilds. There are now 17 and they remain the examining bodies for specialist training.

The Royal College of General Practitioners was not finally formed until 1952. Attempts to establish such a college went back at least a hundred years but were thwarted by external opposition from the surgeons and physicians, as well as by internal arguments among GPs (Hunt 1983). The negotiations over the establishment of the higher training committee for general practice and ongoing debate about whether the MRCGP exam should be a requirement for new GPs and GP trainers highlight continuing internal divisions.

The bodies which oversee postgraduate training – the content of programmes, which posts and institutions are recognised for training – are the nine higher training committees. The Joint Committee on Postgraduate Training for General Practice (JCPTGP) was established as recently as 1975. The joint committees were set up by the royal colleges but include the universities, the Department of Health and others.

The issue as far as general practice is concerned is not that the JCPTGP is not committed to general practice but that they and the other eight higher training committees do not necessarily train their registrars to work with each other. Hospital consultants still give the impression that GPs are doctors who have 'fallen off the ladder' (Moran, 1958).

Hospitals and undergraduate medical schools

While the colleges were examining bodies, in common with other apprenticeship-based systems, they did not provide the teaching or experience. At the beginning of the nineteenth century that role was largely taken by the hospitals. Learning was primarily by 'walking the wards' with evening lectures. After the Medical Act 1858, Medical Schools were established – 12 in London, seven outside.

The Act intended that, on graduation, students should be safe to practise, without further education, in any branch of medicine. After 1867, a pre-clinical and clinical curriculum was prescribed by what became the General Medical Council.

The dominance of hospitals in undergraduate medical education has been almost total. Walton (1997) put it mildly: 'Considerable concern attaches to the obvious fact that medical school teaching is in many ways discrepant from the practice setting where doctors function'.

Sir John Ellis (1979), a distinguished dean of the London Hospital Medical School, wrote: 'Until after World War II, the medical schools of London were superbly equipped to turn schoolboys into GPs by apprenticeship – learning in hospital how to do all that medicine could do outside'. In a lecture about the future of medical education, Ellis presented a picture of Rahere ward at Bart's and said: 'This at the end of the play is what medical education is all about'.

Training is not focused on the largest single destination of graduates. Furthermore hospital doctors are not, generally, taught how to teach and the effectiveness of their teaching is not assessed.

Career choice and who makes a role-model (positive or negative) is much more complex than is often appreciated. However, it is certainly true that hospitals have been well aware that having students was a good way to attract people to work in them. Perhaps it is fear of competing role-models that is the real problem.

Universities

Historically, the place of universities in medical education reflected the physicians' branch of medicine. As 'gentlemen healers' they were expected to study the 'liberal arts' such as the classics, mathematics, philosophy – in different proportions depending on where they studied.

All the free-standing medical schools are now moving into multifaculty universities. This creates opportunities for stronger links with the human and social sciences, schools of education and business schools, which may have much to contribute to medical education. But there is no doubt that there are perceived tensions and threats too. Must doctors be taught by other doctors? Should medical schools employ their own social scientists or should they draw on other faculties? What influence will education specialists have on medical teaching? Humanist or biopsychosocial general practice, in particular, might have much to gain from the multifaculty universities. General practices are small businesses and increased roles in planning and monitoring secondary care might also make them outward-looking, but this perspective may not be shared by all their colleagues.

The deaneries and postgraduate education

Postgraduate medical education was stimulated partly by the desire to train overseas doctors. The model which emerged between the wars was of postgraduate medical schools attached to both universities and hospitals.

Postgraduate education for doctors was first proposed by the Athlone Committee in 1921. It recommended that postgraduate and undergraduate education should not take place in the same medical school (Lister 1993). Although subsequent reports argued that they should, undergraduate and postgraduate education remained organisationally separate.

At the end of World War II the postgraduate medical schools formed a federal structure – the British Postgraduate Medical Federation. The Conference of Deans Postgraduate Medical Education (COPMED), a forum for postgraduate deans to exchange views and determine policy, was also set up after the war. The postgraduate deans of the individual schools were later joined by regional deans. In the mid-1990s, the regional arms of the federation were reconstituted as regional deaneries.

Postgraduate centres became widely established in the 1960s. However, their origins go back to the eighteenth century medical societies. Some of these remained local societies. Others, such as the Royal Society of Medicine, went on to become international academic networks.

The postgraduate centres established in the 1960s were run by 'enthusiastic amateurs' working in 'virtually non-existent time with no training in educational method or curriculum design'. The funding of the centres frequently came from the King Edward Hospital Fund and the Nuffield Provincial Hospitals Fund (Lister 1993). Not until 1991 were clinical tutors paid a sessional payment and not until 1993 did regional advisers in general practice become part of the regional budget for postgraduate medical education.

Education and development at primary care team level

While the system's origins and evolution may help to explain how it is supposed to work, at the level of an individual primary care team, its complexity looks tortuous, particularly when the education and development of other members of the primary care team are taken into account (see Fig.1 opposite).

	Key to Fig. 1
AMSPAR	Association of Medical Secretaries, Practice Managers and Receptionists
CGLI	City and Guilds Institute of London
CPD	Continuing Professional Development
DN	District Nurse
DoH	Department of Health
Educ. Boards	Part of the LIZEI programme, these boards were set up to oversee education in general practice
ENB	English National Board for Nursing
FE	Further Education
FE College	Further Education College
FEFC	Further Education Funding Council
GMC	General Medical Council
HEFC	Higher Education Funding Council
HV	Health Visitor
JCPTGP	Joint Committee on Postgraduate Training for General Practice
RCGP	Royal College of General Practitioners
Reg. Office	Regional Office of NHS Executive
SIFT	Service Increment for Teaching
STA	Specialist Training Authority of the Royal Colleges
VTS	Vocational Training Scheme

Current trends

Medical education may have changed little over the last hundred years but there are a number of reasons why things should be different in the future.

- Demographic changes are going to alter the demand for health care. There are going to be more people who have periods of illness or

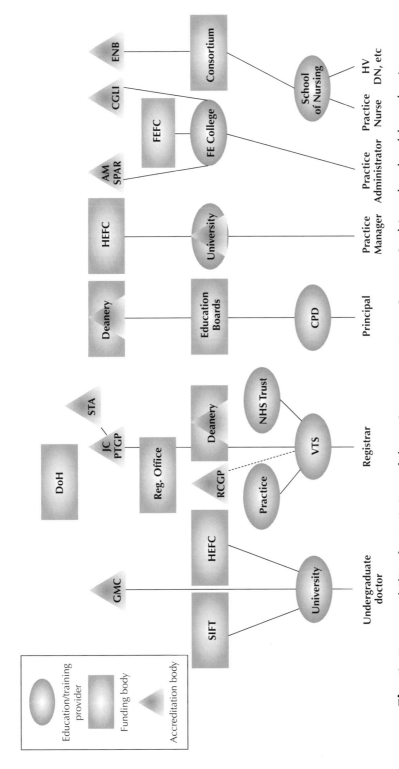

Fig. 1 Responsibility for training of the primary care team in a typical London health authority

impairment, who could be diagnosed, treated, nursed and supported outside hospitals and nursing homes

- Expectations of what professionals can and should do will change. Users are less likely to accept that 'doctor knows best' without at least some evidence that doctors are updating their practice

- There will be changes in patterns of public and private spending and expectations about how services are provided. There have been dramatic shifts in provision and financial responsibility for continuing care in the last ten years. The Government has signalled its intention to make further changes in a series of White and Green Papers. General practice will be profoundly affected

- A specific challenge will be to develop the necessary skills, knowledge and attitudes to face the organisational changes brought about by primary care groups, primary care trusts and health improvement programmes

- The GMC's new competence procedures and new arrangements for clinical governance will also have an impact on the medical profession. There will be internal pressures for change. In documents such as *Tomorrow's Doctors,* the GMC (1993) has set out its vision of what medical education should look like and, through its powers of inspection and recognition, can strongly influence what happens. The recommendations in *Tomorrow's Doctors* included: reducing the burden of factual knowledge; promoting learning and self-education through curiosity, exploration and critical evaluation of evidence; employing learning systems informed by modern educational theory

- Modern education theory reinforces the importance of self-directed learning, learning from peers, reflective practice, distance-learning techniques and resources (computers, television) as the alternatives to the traditional hospital or university campus

- Radically different visions of the purpose of general practice may emerge. Primary care, including general practice, is established as an appropriate site for delivering services and a workplace for those people who do it – a 'locus'. It is increasingly recognised as a more appropriate place to prevent ill health, diagnose and manage – a 'focus'.

A more radical extension of treating the community as both a locus and a focus is to recognise the role of the public in defining needs and in identifying and implementing solutions. The really significant improvements in life expectancy are the result of economic, social and environmental improvements, not health services (Wilkinson 1996).

The 'down side' of a largely free and universal national health service is that it may have turned the population from being active producers of their health, identifying their health care needs and demanding the conditions which promote health and well-being (Hart 1988). If there is to be any shift towards the public as producers of health, it will require a dramatic change in the way that health care workers are trained, so that they can genuinely be advocates enhancing choice and control, particularly of the most vulnerable individuals and populations. Changing the way doctors are trained would be central to improving the health of the population in this model.

Whatever the model of primary care, there are going to be some central questions for the future. The answers to these questions will be informed by the values that motivate the key players.

Questions and values

What is education for?

This historical outline has identified that education and training provision has not always had improvements in service in general practice as its central focus. The present Government emphasises equity and health improvement, and demonstrable links to standards and quality in services are likely to be required. More user-sensitive, less fragmented services are part of the vision.

The themes are explored in Chapter 2, which looks at the principles underlying education and training in the NHS and Chapter 5, which considers issues of measuring quality in general practice. Chapter 6 describes the role of patients as educators and the nursing and wider primary care team perspectives thereby making the case for a holistic, user-centred education.

Who is to be educated?

'Lifelong learning' is identified by the Government as a requirement for a 'first class' health service (DoH 1998). It is clear that education in and for general practice will span undergraduate medical students (and increasing numbers of nurses) through to long-established GPs. Non-principals and other practice staff will also need to be trained. The reviews of the LIZEI programmes in Chapter 3 demonstrate that training can reach all practitioners, not just a select few, if it is set up on the right lines.

Interprofessional education is no longer the enthusiasm of a few. It is now widely seen as an essential priority, not just for established practitioners but from undergraduate and initial training onwards.

How and where are people to be educated?

General practice will be a focus of medical education. To release the potential of general practice to be a locus of education requires planning and resources. General practice as a learning environment is discussed in Chapter 4.

Who will plan and who will deliver education?

The present Government places a great deal of emphasis on partnerships – including with users – and bringing down barriers between agencies. This represents a shift from the more individualistic ideology of the previous administration. Shared responsibility for the whole 'region' of education and training for primary care, rather than a 'carve-up' or shift of responsibility between different agencies, is likely to be demanded. This will embrace professional bodies (such as the RCGP, LMCs, nursing bodies), educational bodies, health authorities, trusts and primary care groups, patients and practising GPs, nurses and others. The various perspectives discussed in Chapter 7 illustrate some of the implications of this.

How will education be judged?

Educational performance is likely to be judged increasingly on end-of-course assessment of participants. More attention will be paid to ensuring that the trainers are skilled and are using effective educational methods. However, throughout this book it is stressed that ultimately the results of education should be judged on the impact it has on service delivery. This is the major challenge for education-service partnerships.

References

Bosanquet N (1996). Primary care – how will the revolution impact on trusts. In: Fitzhugh (ed.) *Directory of NHS Trusts*. London: HCIS

Brackenbury H (1935). *Doctor and Patient*. London: Hodder and Stoughton,

CCCS (Centre for Contemporary Cultural Studies) (1981). *Education Group; Unpopular Education; Schooling and Social Democracy*. London: Hutchinson

Department of Health (1997). *The New NHS – Modern, Dependable*. London: The Stationery Office, Cm 3807

Department of Health (1998). *A First Class Service – Quality in the new NHS*. London: The Stationery Office

Downie R, Charlton B (1992) .*The Making of a Doctor; Medical Education in Theory and Practice*. Oxford: OUP

Ellis J (1979). *London Hospital Medical Club 1785–1985: The Story of England's first medical school*. LHMC

Ellis J (1979). Medical Education in London. Schornstein Lecture. St Bartholomew's Medical College, London

Engel G (1992). The biopsychosocial model and medical education. *New England Journal of Medicine* 30(13):802–5

Engel G (1994). The need for a new medical model: a challenge for biomedicine. *Science* 196(4286):129–36

Fraser RC (1987). *Clinical Method – A General Practice Approach*. London: Butterworth & Heinemann

GMC (1993). *Tomorrow's Doctors*. London: General Medical Council

GMSC (1996). *Defining Core Services*. London: BMA

Hart JT (1988). *A New Kind of Doctor*. London: Merlin

Hindmarsh J *et al.* (1998). Are vocationally trained GPs better GPs? A review of research designs and outcomes. *Medical Education* 32:244–54

Horder J, Swift G (1979). The history of vocational training for general practice. *Journal of the Royal College of GPs* 29:24–32

Hunt J (1983). In: Fry J, Hunt J, Pinsent R (eds). *A History of the Royal College of General Practitioners*. Lancaster: MTP Press

Honigsbaum F (1979). *The Division in British Medicine*. London: Kogan Page

Lewis J (1997). The GP contract under the NHS. In: Ellis N, Chisolm J. *Making Sense of the Red Book*. 3rd edition, Abingdon: Radcliffe

Lister J (1993). *Postgraduate Medical Education*. Nuffield Provincial Hospitals Trust

McCormick (1992). In: Downie R, Charlton B, op. cit.

Moran (1958) quoted by Toon op. cit.

Oswald NT (1989). Why not base medical education in general practice? *Lancet* 2:148–9

Perry P (1976). *The Evolution of British Manpower Policy* (published by the author).

Richards P (1993). *Learning Medicine*. London: BMJ Publishing

Saddington JA (1992). Learner experience: a rich resource for learning. In: Mulligan, Griffith (eds). *Empowerment through Experiential Learning*. London: Kogan Page

Schön D (1991). *The Reflective Practitioner*. Aldershot: Arena

Simon B (1974). The politics of educational reform, 1920–1940. In: Lawrence and Wishart. *Education and the Labour Movement 1920–1940*. London: Lawrence and Wishart

Toon P (1994). *What is Good General Practice?* Occasional Paper no. 65 RCGP

Tooth D, Tonge K, McManus I (1989). Anxiety and study methods in pre-clinical students: causal relationships to examine performance. *Medical Education* 23:416–21

Vuori H (1996). In: Atun R, Lang H (eds). *What Is Good Primary Care?* London: Imperial College
Walton H (1997). In: McLachlan G (ed). *Medical Education and Medical Care; A Scottish-American Symposium.* Oxford: Oxford University Press

Weil S, McGill I (eds) (1989). *Making Sense of Experiential Learning.* Milton Keynes: Open University Press

Weatherall D (1993) (Professor of Medicine at Oxford). In: Lowry S (ed). *Medical Education.* London: BMJ Publishing Group

Whitehouse C, Roland M, Campion P (1997). *Teaching Medicine in the Community – A Guide for Undergraduate Education.* Oxford: OUP

This chapter draws on work in progress by Dr Anita Berlin whose help is gratefully acknowledged as is the advice of Dr John Horder.

Chapter 2

Education and training in the NHS: principles and process

Steve Gillam, Charles Easmon and Philip Leech

KEY POINTS

- Adult learning methods are increasingly replacing traditional didactic approaches to the training of doctors

- The CMO's report on continuing professional development in general practice stresses the importance of properly co-ordinated practice-based plans

- The New NHS White Paper and the advent of clinical governance place new demands on primary care professionals and those responsible for their education and training

- Though still developing, education consortia with their broad-based membership are appropriate bodies to commission training in support of these demands

- If properly co-ordinated, the system of national education levies (SIFT, MADEL and NMET) together with R&D funds provides the wherewithal to develop primary care. The different funding streams have yet to be devoted to maximum effect

The purpose of medical education

The ultimate purpose of medical education is to improve the care of patients in the NHS. Education should be enjoyable and fulfilling in its own right: it is not occupational therapy for health professionals. Medical knowledge is expanding at an exponential rate. Doctors are struggling to keep up with this information deluge and Giraud (1993) has gloomily calculated that clinicians who read one article per day given the number of medical journals published, fall 55 centuries behind in their reading within a year!

This is not an excuse for low standards and an inability to keep up. Doctors can only ever attempt to learn a portion of what is available to be learned: much is soon forgotten and much of what is retained becomes obsolete. The challenge is to match the relevant knowledge to the particular characteristics of the patient presenting. A duty of care has to be underpinned by engagement with modern, authoritative opinion, and an understanding of new technologies and methods of delivering care. Clinicians can no longer simply absorb a myriad of facts. They must understand how to apply learning in clinical situations and use information technology to support it. The best ways of learning, of presenting knowledge and promoting understanding are changing. They also vary between individuals and in different situations.

Education and training, research and development (R&D), and service provision form three overlapping systems. They should constantly interact but all too often education has been seen as remote from service activity. The day-to-day pressures of life in the Health Service do not engender a naturally reflective culture. Education, training and research help inject that critical element. The starting point for the development of these three systems should be a clear understanding of the population's health and health care needs. What research is required, what services should be provided and how do we develop the skilled staff to deliver them? These three systems should no longer occupy separate professional boxes. The advent of a national R&D strategy and alterations to the way education is funded are helping to change that.

What do doctors need to learn?

Iona Heath has elegantly outlined the generic roles of a GP: interpreting a patient's story, guarding against overmedicalisation and witnessing a patient's suffering in the absence of other help (Heath, 1995). A first priority is learning about fundamental clinical skills: history taking and examination. The second priority is to understand the natural history of disease: how it presents, progresses, varies and evolves. The third, especially in general practice, is that you must learn to question how disease may affect the individual patient. Learning about people, not patients, and about health, not illness, is the fourth fundamental.

Doctors learn in many different ways. They learn by telling tales – discussing cases and relaying anecdotes. They learn by looking back and reflecting. Increasingly, they learn through new interactive information technologies. *The new NHS* White Paper makes a strong commitment to networking, to the development of electronic data interchange and decision support. New software programmes such as WAX, Prodigy and Best Answers are the forerunners of tools that will transform medical practice in the next century. Prodigy, for example, is decision support software developed to aid the act of prescribing. It is now expanding to include audit loops, referral and investigation queries. In future, it may interrogate clinical records and accommodate the previous prescribing behaviour of the GP using it.

The 1997 education White Paper embraces the underlying principles of lifelong learning in a learning society (see Box 1).

BOX 1 PREREQUISITES FOR A LEARNING SOCIETY

A culture where values and processes of learning are suffused throughout

A political system that values participative democracy and active citizenship

Provision of learning should be responsive to the needs of the whole community

Learning processes should be active and participative

Learning should be aimed at self-development

Assessment and qualification should encourage achievement, not be primarily for selection

Learning skills and knowledge should be seen by stakeholders as central to success

This is not mere Blairite rhetoric. The notion of a learning society where the principles of continuing development suffuse all work environments is a powerful one. However, for health professionals it is also challenging. It implies a willingness to meet the public's ever more sophisticated requirements for information and to share decision-making. In the Health Service, as in society at large, people can be turned off. The educational process may be seen as irrelevant or regimented. Learning is rarely a product of compulsion. Professional obligations provide a more powerful imperative than contractual ones. Health professionals share accountability for the money spent on the educational process.

Education as preparation for the unknown

Education is perhaps best defined as 'preparation for the unknown'. Health professionals have to be equipped to manage continuous change. This challenge goes beyond continually updating clinical skills to cope with new knowledge. Professional development needs to be linked to wider practice development, which in turn may reflect changing patients' needs. *The new NHS* White Paper underlines this. The move to a primary care-centred NHS is a belated response to longer-term demographic imperatives. Today's burden of chronic diseases is best managed in the community.

Training and development systems in general practice have hardly begun to equip GPs for some of the responsibilities they face today as commissioners of care. Doctors are supremely opportunistic in attaining career end points ('Where do I want to go and how might I best get there?') but they are not necessarily able to identify longer-term needs. The London Initiative Zone Education Incentive (LIZEI) programme has helped to remedy this. Health improvement programmes should provide the planning framework into which local education strategies can slot. As primary care groups (PCGs) evolve, the education/service partnership will need to be rethought in support of areas such as clinical governance.

The most obvious gaps in *The new NHS* White Paper concern the developmental underpinnings for the massive organisational changes proposed. Staff wastage is in some ways an even bigger problem in general practice than in trusts and health authorities. Many doctors are leaving the service prematurely and little more than a quarter of graduates choose this career option. For nurses the recruitment problem has reached crisis proportions. Currently, many experienced practice managers are thought to be departing the service. The abolition of fundholding is likely to accelerate this. The traditional response has been to pour more water into the leaking bucket – to train more people. We have only recently begun to try to mend the bucket – to increase our understanding of why staff leave and to address their concerns.

The CMO's report on continuing professional development

The requirement for different approaches to education at different stages of a health professional's career is echoed in the conclusions of the Chief Medical Officer (CMO)'s review of continuing professional development in general practice. He identified several problems with the current system (see Box 2).

BOX 2 PROBLEMS IDENTIFIED IN CMO REVIEW

- Lack of clear and coherent planning:
  – in provision of educational opportunities
  – by practitioners in making use of current programmes

- Practices and practitioners find it difficult to set clear goals

- Absence of facilitation of joint learning

- PGEA fails to demonstrate convincing benefits for patient care

- Too much activity is didactic, uniprofessional and top-down

- Too little activity is participative

- Hardly any involves the practice team

- Meetings often demonstrate sectoral interests and are biased towards secondary care

---

Moving on from PGEA

The postgraduate education accreditation (PGEA) system provides direct financial incentives for GPs to attend ten days of educational activity per year. It successfully places 'bums on seats' but is fatally flawed. The evidence suggests that traditional didactic approaches to learning are ineffective in changing behaviour. Little forethought is required from participants regarding their practices' or their patients' needs.

Classically, a single partner goes off on a course to learn more about something that they know much about already. They return brimful with enthusiasm to a practice that is as unreceptive as ever to their new ideas. Harmony in general practice can be difficult enough to maintain at the best of times; this kind of educational experience can be positively damaging. Nor is educational activity matched to the particular learning needs of the participants. Education needs to encompass audit, effectiveness and relevant research. A properly co-ordinated educational process needs to embrace the whole primary health care team; by extension more of this activity should be practice-based.

The practice professional development plan is therefore at the centre of the CMO's recommendations. It should be based on service development plans that have matched practice objectives to their patients' needs. The process should be professionally led and monitored through peer review. It should embrace personal, clinical and organisational development.

Clinical governance in the 'new NHS'

The advent of clinical governance should simultaneously promote quality and accountability. *The new NHS* White Paper outlined the principles and processes involved (see Box 3).

Clinical governance places responsibilities and expectations on both individuals and organisations for the delivery of high-quality health care. Individuals will be expected to work within explicit standards of professional performance, engaging in continuing professional development and acknowledging the strategic objectives of the organisation they work within. On the other hand, organisations – trusts and PCGs – will have responsibilities to support training and development, provide access to information, feeding back data that help clinicians assess their performance.

BOX 3   PRINCIPLES OF CLINICAL GOVERNANCE

- A quality organisation will ensure that:

- quality improvement processes (e.g. clinical audit) are in place and integrated with the quality programme for the organisation as a whole

- leadership skills are developed at clinical team level

- evidence-based practice is in day-to-day use with the infrastructure to support it

- good practice, ideas and innovations (which have been evaluated) are systematically disseminated within and outside the organisation

- clinical risk reduction programmes of a high standard are in place

- adverse events are detected and openly investigated and the lessons learned promptly applied

- lessons for clinical practice are systematically learned from complaints made by patients

- problems of poor clinical performance are recognised at an early stage and dealt with to prevent harm to patients

- all professional development programmes reflect the principles of clinical governance

- the quality of data gathered to monitor clinical care is itself of a high standard

Source: *The new NHS* (1987)

The development of clinical governance within PCGs presents major challenges. As in trusts, lead executives will be held accountable for the quality of care their constituents deliver. GPs do not see themselves as their brothers' or sisters' keeper within a practice, let alone within a practice grouping. Special individuals with advanced facilitation skills will be required to engender the trust needed to change interpractice relations in this way. A particular test of clinical governance will be the extent to which it addresses the problems at the lower end of the quality spectrum – those that have always been 'hardest to reach'.

The National Institute of Clinical Excellence (NICE) will provide national service frameworks and the guidance needed to implement these. The Commission for Health Improvement (CHI) will advance the new performance management framework. PCGs will be contributing to their local health improvement programmes. This panoply of new arrangements should both advance and target practice-based learning. They will also paradoxically create new learning needs. How, for example, are GPs to contribute to their local health improvement programmes?

The new NHS White Paper thus places a heavy burden on those with responsibilities for educating and training GPs. On balance, the opportunities outweigh the threats. The practice is the key learning environment for the immediate future.

Funding streams

The NHS spends around £1.5bn on the education and training of clinical professionals. This is levied from financial allocations to health authorities. Larger NHS institutions like hospital trusts can also use a proportion of the money they derive from clinical contracts on staff development. Hitherto, for smaller organisations such as general practices this has been difficult. PCGs, on the other hand, may be able to form new partnerships. Table 1 illustrates how these levies totalling £390m are distributed in one area, North Thames.

Service increment for teaching (SIFT)

SIFT supports the demonstrated excess costs to an institution of teaching medical students. Eighty per cent of SIFT is linked to the long-term infrastructure costs of such support facilities, 20 per cent to the more variable costs linked to actual student numbers (clinical placements). Each clinical placement represents one student in training on site for a full academic year. Each attracts just over £8000 per year and their distribution is decided by each medical school.

General practice only became eligible for SIFT payments in 1996/7. To date, this has largely been limited to clinical placement funding. In 1998/99, some facilities funding will be applied to general practice. This

Table 1 National NHS levies

	Non Medical Education and Training (NMET)	Postgraduate Medical and Dental Education (MADEL)	Service Increment for Teaching (SIFT) R&D	R&D
Levy				
Staff groups	Nurses, midwives, professions allied to medicine, clinical scientists	Doctors and dentists in postgraduate training	Medical/dental undergraduates	All groups of NHS staff engaged in R&D
Budget responsibility	Regional office, education consortia	Deans of postgraduate medicine through regional offices	Medical schools, NHS trusts, regional offices	NHS trusts and regional offices
1998–99 North Thames	£150m	£120m	£120m	£203m

is needed if general practice is to become the main locus for teaching clinical skills, attitudes and behaviour. Nearly half of all medical students become GPs and this development is in line with the GMC's recommendation in *Tomorrow's Doctors* for more community-based teaching. Without proper support from SIFT, the necessary curricular change cannot be sustained. In London SIFT needs to be used to support what the LIZEI programme has helped to establish.

Medical and dental education levy (MADEL)

This levy supports postgraduate medical and dental education (PGMDE), including the provision of education, library and study leave for hospital-based trainees. In general practice, MADEL covers the PGMDE structure of the directors of postgraduate general practice education, their network of associates and vocational training scheme course organisers. In general practice, the education system is directly involved in continuing medical education (CME) for GP principals, through the GP tutors and PGEA.

Although SIFT and MADEL are separate and funds cannot be switched around at regional level, there is scope for closer working between the two. The common ground is the training practice. If this covers both undergraduate and postgraduate medical education, a practice can receive support from both levies. With the greater involvement of general practice at the pre-registration house officer level, there is the possibility of a real continuum of general practice involvement in medical education – from student to GP principal. A higher profile for GP teacher role models could have an impact on career choice and recruitment to general practice.

R&D

The first round of bids for R&D portfolio and tasked-linked funding has just been completed. A number of primary care networks have been supported. Many of the practices will also be undergraduate and/or postgraduate teaching practices with clinical placements from a range of professions. These are training practices that blur the divisions between R&D and education.

The national R&D budget is £425m. This is divided into two budgets:

- Budget One (the Culyer stream) is for NHS providers and amounts to a total of £350m. For North Thames (1998/99) there is a total of some £196m and of this about £1m goes to primary care. The rest is awarded to NHS provider trusts engaged in research activity
- Budget Two totals £75m nationally for commissioned research projects. North Thames region receives £6.5m of this.

Non-medical education and training (NMET) levy

NMET covers the pre- and post-registration training of professions, including nursing, midwifery and health visiting, occupational therapy, physiotherapy, radiography, clinical psychology, clinical scientists, pharmacy, speech and language therapy, dietetics, chiropody and dental support staff. Nationally, the NMET levy is just over £800m.

All the levies mentioned so far are national money but resources are also available locally. For example, GP educators may receive assistance from health authorities, from drug companies and other sources. The service needs to be much more imaginative in the way cash is apportioned to support development beyond traditional clinical education. For example, the NMET budget has a special remit for personal development not limited to any particular staff group. This has not yet been taken up. Much hinges on the new education consortia.

Education consortia

An education consortium consists of employers of NHS-trained clinical professionals (not limited to the NHS) and health authority and GP commissioners of health care. Its purpose is to use NMET funds to purchase appropriate high-quality education for clinical professionals through contracts with higher education, to carry out workforce planning and to determine the extent of training needed. This is to satisfy both local and national needs. Consortia also have a responsibility for personal and organisational management and need to link with postgraduate deans and medical workforce advisory groups so that a more integrated approach to workforce planning can be developed.

Consortia are dominated by acute trusts. Primary care representation through health authorities and GPs is still weak. GMS workforce planning is a health authority responsibility, although this is now being brought into some consortia. Primary care education boards are one way of linking consortia with primary care more effectively. *The New NHS* should provide a stimulus for consortia to give primary care a higher priority. Consortia do represent a major part of the local health care economy and can play a significant role in driving forward primary care education.

Again taking North Thames as an example, there are eight education consortia of which seven assumed full financial contractual independence from 1 April 1998. They control the bulk of the region's £150m NMET allocation. Their influence extends beyond the NHS into social services and the voluntary and independent sectors. Though still at a formative stage, the wide cross-representation from service institutions gives consortia greater leverage and broader insight into health professionals' training needs. They effectively control the delivery of education at both undergraduate and post-basic qualification level for those who are not doctors and dentists. This is arguably of greater significance to local health economies than the national supply of doctors and dentists. The continuing emphasis on primary care-based commissioning places an obvious imperative on consortia to anticipate demands from this sector. Consortia are young, fragile organisations that will need time to properly assume their responsibilities. Collaboration does not come easily to those who have been previously encouraged to compete to provide education.

Moving forward

The LIZEI programme ended in March 1998. It has stimulated an immense amount of activity in four areas: undergraduate education in general practice; innovations in vocational and post-vocational training; academic fellowships and support schemes; and general educational opportunities (with the necessary locum support) for established GPs.

In the last category, the emphasis on encouraging personal development plans should in turn link with practice development plans. This planned development contrasts with the opportunistic learning that characterises

PGEA. The amount of activity generated by LIZEI has outstripped the original targets. Early findings of an evaluation of the effectiveness of the programme, commissioned through the national R&D programme and undertaken by a team from Nottingham University, are considered in the next chapter.

The challenge for those who have managed and benefited from LIZEI is to take forward its successes. *The new NHS* provides further opportunities for partnership between education and service in primary care, not only in the traditional areas of clinical professional education, but in the broader areas linking personal and organisational development. The challenges of clinical governance and PCG formation require a coherent programme of development to help the various professional groups respond effectively.

References

Chief Medical Officer (1998). A *Review of Continuing Professional Development in General Practice*. London: Department of Health

General Medical Council (1993). *Tomorrow's Doctors*. London: GMC

Giraud A (1992). Uncertainty in medicine – can it be reduced? *Quality in Health Care*, 1:150–1

Haines A, Jones R (1994). Implementing findings of research. *British Medical Journal* 308(14):88–92

Heath I (1995). *The Mystery of General Practice*. London: Nuffield Provincial Hospitals Trust

Chapter 3

Lessons from LIZEI

Isobel Bowler, Roland Petchey and Roger Murphy

KEY POINTS

- A substantial programme of continuing professional development for general practice, based on the experience of LIZEI, requires meticulous planning

- Between 12 and 24 months lead-in time is needed to set up infrastructure, a range of needs assessment tools and an evaluation system

- To develop learning opportunities a partnership is needed between practitioners, health authorities, academic departments, colleagues in the primary care team as well as people with a broader understanding of adult learning. Education needs to be inclusive of non-principals

- The planning framework should place benefits to patients foremost and, in that context, the needs of individual practitioners. It should include locum costs and protected time for education, and it should extend beyond three years

- Four different patterns of use of LIZEI funding were identified: academic trainees; big bidders; accumulators; and non-bidders. These reflected different learning styles and levels of educational development.

Between April 1995 and March 1998 GPs in the primary care development zone in London (the London Initiative Zone or LIZ) benefited from large-scale investment in continuing medical education. The LIZ Educational Incentives (LIZEI) programme was conceived as an addition to the primary care development initiative for London set out in response to the Tomlinson report on London's health services. Against a background of concern about the inner London GP workforce, the programme was intended to address the recruitment, retention and refreshment of GPs. LIZEI had four key objectives:

- to extend and provide more effective undergraduate medical education in the community
- to pilot innovations in vocational training for general practice
- to provide career development opportunities for GPs in education and research
- to promote professional development for existing GP principals.

Over the three years of the LIZEI programme, £34m was made available for these four areas of activity. Of this approximately half has been spent on support and provision of professional development for the 2500 GP principals within the LIZ.

Detailed information on overall patterns of activity within the LIZEI programme is available in its annual report (NHSE 1997). This chapter will focus upon a central element – the programmes of professional development for existing GP principals. However, it is important to note that there is considerable overlap between the four objectives identified above. For instance, the programmes targeting community-based undergraduate medical education have necessarily also involved professional development opportunities for GP principals. Thus, in the North Thames area of the LIZ more than 400 GPs have received training on teaching undergraduates.

Organisation of LIZEI

The programme was co-ordinated by two regional steering groups (for North Thames and South Thames). Their membership included the key stakeholders in the programme:

- the NHS Executive
- health authorities
- university departments of general practice
- Thames Postgraduate Medical and Dental Education
- local medical committees (LMCs).

In each health authority area an education board was set up to plan and administer the local programme. The composition of the education board varied across the 12 LIZ areas, but typically it included:

- the health authority
- medical audit advisory group (MAAG)
- local medical committee
- GP tutors
- GP course organisers
- the postgraduate dean (or representative)
- the undergraduate department of general practice
- representatives of local GPs.

In some places the boards also included representatives of other primary health care professionals and nurse education. The regional steering groups also funded programmes of academic support from the eight London university departments of general practice, the University of Westminster and the two North Thames postgraduate deaneries.

The key tasks in planning and implementing the LIZEI programme locally were:

- needs assessment (both professional development needs and service needs)
- informing GPs about the programme
- supporting GPs in identifying their needs and planning their educational activities
- commissioning education and other activities funded under the programme
- scrutinising GPs' requests for funding for self-selected educational activity
- reflecting on progress and planning future activity.

As part of our external evaluation activity we facilitated an evaluation workshop with local representatives from the 12 LIZ areas. These were people who had been involved in planning and delivering local programmes. They singled out the education board structure as having been very valuable. It had provided the impetus to bring together service and education, and had helped to make better links between undergraduate and postgraduate general practice. In some of the 12 LIZ areas, boards were highly successful and it was decided to continue beyond the LIZEI funding, collaborating with other groups to cover more of the primary health care team (depending on the future arrangements for GP professional development).

Elsewhere, however, boards had been less successful, even dysfunctional. This was attributed to pre-existing poor relationships between organisations and individuals, or power imbalances between different partners on the boards. A difficulty in determining board membership was reconciling representation of all stakeholders with achieving a functional group which was not too large. One solution to this problem was to have a large board with all stakeholders represented, with a smaller executive group bringing proposals to the larger group. For this to work there needed to be a good relationship of trust between stakeholders. Where there is no clear structure, there is a danger that some partners feel excluded from decision-making.

Implementing LIZEI

Health authorities took different approaches to the LIZEI implementation in the 12 LIZ areas. In all 12 they were responsible for administering the local budget and were represented on the education boards, often at director level. However, the way in which they became involved in implementing the programmes varied. Money was available for LIZEI co-ordinators and the type of person employed ranged from administrative staff to a GP with an educational background. The role of this person ranged from predominantly administrative (managing budgets) to being involved at all levels including 'hands on' implementation. Some health authorities ran the LIZEI programme with existing staff (e.g. primary care provider development manager). Others made use of health authority-employed staff in outposted units (e.g. the GP link office in Croydon which already had a role in facilitating educational activities for GPs), or staff funded through education boards (e.g. MAAG staff). In a few health authorities there was little involvement beyond financial management and membership of the education board, with the major role being delegated to GP tutors. The level of involvement was determined to an extent by the background of the staff in post at the time, and by whether there were senior staff from the former family health services authority working in the health authority.

Relationships

The relationship between health authorities and GPs is often a sensitive one. On one side, GPs have historically resisted external infringements of their independent contractor status. On the other, HAs have until recently had little experience of dealing with GPs. The role of health authorities in professional development is by no means clear – and some of the tensions which have arisen between GPs on the ground and health authorities/education boards stem from this contradiction between monitoring and coaching roles. Staff in academic units suggested that some of the activities they provided as part of the programme were popular with GPs who did not want to become too closely involved with their local health authority.

The organisational flux and rapid staff turnover which resulted from the round of DHA mergers preceding the creation of new health authorities in April 1996 (one year into the LIZEI programme) may have further compromised the capacity of some HAs to respond rapidly to this new management task. HAs which were already operating as health commissions and health agencies prior to 1996 had more management energy to apply to the LIZEI than those which were in the midst of reorganisation during the three-year programme. Health authorities with staff from the old FHSA had the advantage of good local knowledge of GPs and a history of working with them.

There were some tensions inherent in the LIZEI programme. First there was a tension between personal and professional development. Related to this was the tension between GP 'wants' (self-defined) and GP 'needs' (as perceived by an outsider). Finally, there was a conflict between the needs of the service (as defined by health needs assessment and health authority agendas) and the needs/wants of GPs to the exclusion of other professional groups such as nurses in primary care. Boards were conscious of the need to ensure that resources were not monopolised by practices which were already well organised, well resourced and well versed in finding their way round the system. They facilitated applications from less well-developed practices. At the same time, it was recognised that the law of diminishing returns might apply also to the investment of time and effort into a practice. The large amounts of money available for the three years of the programme meant that there was generally enough money to fund most of the programmes and activities different groups wanted. This has minimised the tensions between service need and GP need, and between needs, wants and demands. In longer-term programmes with less generous funding, these tensions are likely to be more apparent.

Funding

The nature of the LIZEI funding created problems for those planning and implementing the programmes. There was difficulty reconciling the need for long-term reform of continuing professional development and short-term investment of large amounts of money. There was little time to plan the programme in the first year, and education board members (especially HAs who were responsible for the budget) reported a 'pressure to spend' which led them to implement programmes in advance of the needs assessment and strategic planning work which should have preceded them.

Where staff needed to be recruited, especially in academic units, it was difficult to get appropriate people in post quickly enough – particularly when the most that could be offered was a three-year contract. At the other end of the programme, there was an inevitable running-down of activity in anticipation of the end of funding. Staff with insecure contracts left early in order to ensure continuity of employment. Much knowledge and expertise was lost to the NHS.

Good practice in continuing professional development

The LIZEI has, in contrast with the PGEA system, fostered a much broader and more innovative programme of activity. There has been great diversity in content. Although clinical skills have continued to be a major focus, other topics have included training in practice management, especially IT training, managing staff, team-building activity, learning self-care (e.g. stress management) and developing teaching, training and tutoring skills. GPs have also had the opportunity to study for the MRCGP (Member of the Royal College of General Practitioners) and a range of diplomas. Some have completed master's degree courses, and even doctoral research. Professional development has been delivered in a variety of ways in addition to the lecture. These have included:

- self-directed learning groups
- peer-supported learning
- mentoring
- individual study
- distance learning
- research
- practice-based learning
- clinical attachments to hospital specialists.

The duration of educational activities was also highly variable. Although the majority of activities were of less than three days, there was a significant investment in longer-term activities, e.g. one day per week for several months, a monthly half-day meeting throughout the LIZEI funding period. Some GPs took career breaks of up to a year to follow a master's course, or other structured activity.

Above all, the LIZEI has given GPs a range of new learning experiences, and helped them to consider alternatives to their traditional approach to CPD, particularly more reflective styles of adult learning. The uptake of the educational opportunities (over 75 per cent of the GPs eligible) shows that GPs are not averse to this. The particular learning strategies adopted by GPs in London are discussed in detail below. It should be noted that levels of funding under LIZEI were very generous, with 100 per cent reimbursement of course fees and travel expenses, and over 100 per cent reimbursement of locum costs. There were some difficulties in finding sufficient locums to provide cover, although as the programme progressed strategies for helping GPs obtain cover were developed. For example, some of the academic unit programmes, such as career breaks, included vocationally trained assistants to cover participating GPs. However, there were some GPs who found it extremely difficult to hand over the practice to another doctor. Securing protected time should not be underestimated as a barrier to GPs engaging in innovative methods of professional development.

Needs assessment

On the whole (with some exceptions, such as Brent and Harrow) no health authorities had professional development strategies covering GP principals. At least one education board commissioned an academic department of general practice to conduct a systematic analysis of the educational and professional needs of the GPs in their patch. Its findings confirmed earlier studies. GPs (before LIZEI) were somewhat conventional and pragmatic in their approach to CME, and were primarily motivated to further clinical study by the identification of a gap in knowledge. Few were likely to plan their education in the long term or to discuss it with others. Elsewhere, needs assessment was more ad hoc. Often it was combined with informing GPs about the new opportunities available and helping them to identify their professional development needs and wants on an individual basis (frequently through visits to the GP in their practice). GP tutors often took on this role, although in some places local GPs were involved as local educational advisers or GP visitors.

Activity to address service needs

In some areas education boards themselves commissioned LIZEI activities to address particular service needs which HAs had identified. A common example is dermatology training to give GPs the necessary clinical skills to conduct investigation and preliminary diagnosis and so reduce referrals. Elsewhere a perceived failure to address teenagers' sexual health needs has led to a family planning and sexual health training project. In one area local GPs were given the opportunity to bid for funding to run local projects for their peers.

Outreach activity – GP visiting

It was common across the LIZ area for GPs to be offered a visit by the education board. The visitor was generally another GP. There are examples of educational facilitators who did not have a medical background taking on this role (e.g. the non-GP tutor for GPs in Enfield and Haringey). The following functions of GP visits were identified:

- to build up knowledge about the local GPs and their needs – this could then be fed into the development of appropriate professional development programmes locally
- to publicise the LIZEI programme
- to encourage uptake
- to disseminate information about local educational opportunities
- to help GPs develop a personal education or development plan
- to help GPs review their progress against their plan and facilitate their continued development.

A key condition for the success of this approach was that appropriate visitors were selected, and in areas where they had been recruited locally this was felt to have been mutually beneficial. The visitors themselves received training, remuneration and reimbursement of locum costs. Above all, it was essential that visitors should not be identified with 'authority' or with performance monitoring. Visitors have reported that they commonly encountered GPs with extremely low morale and in some cases with a need for significant levels of personal and emotional support, over and above their professional development.

We have found cases where GPs decided to leave general practice as a result of examining their situation with the LIZEI visitor. It was considered vital that visiting GPs were themselves supported so that they did not feel isolated or become 'ground down' by the low morale among some of the GPs they visited.

Portfolio learning

LIZEI has encouraged GPs to identify personal and professional learning goals, and address these with a portfolio of activities. The learning plan has to encompass more than narrowly defined job-related training and development, and a reflective portfolio approach was seen as having important strengths:

- different styles of learning can be accommodated
- different levels of participation are possible
- it is owned by the GP (or other participant)
- it allows a 'bottom-up' influence on the agenda

- individuals are measured against their own learning plan and their 'portfolio' reflects their achievement
- the process of reflection means that the learning plans can inform the design and delivery of future programmes, so feeding into further needs assessment
- it is not reliant on special funding.

However, problems were also identified. For the majority of GPs, it involved an approach to learning which was radically different from the one which they had become accustomed to at medical school and subsequently. It could therefore be perceived as threatening. There could also be problems sustaining motivation and finding protected time.

Innovation in delivery of professional development

Across the LIZ a variety of projects have experimented with a range of facilitation styles in small-group and individual learning. These have ranged from self-directed groups, facilitated by the participating GPs themselves, through GP-tutor-facilitated groups, to groups focusing on attaining the MRCGP. Groups have the following additional benefits:

- they can reduce personal and professional isolation, particularly among GPs in single- and two-handed practices
- self-directed groups can be continued without special funding, although participation would be lower without paid locum cover
- they can provide personal and pastoral support beyond the explicit educational purpose of the group.

However, the schemes were organisationally very complex, the groups needed significant facilitation input to begin with, and withdrawal of the facilitation support could be difficult to negotiate. Where there was not a specific objective (e.g. the MRCGP), the impossibility of separating out personal and professional development could lead to problems in specifying the objectives of the groups. Such schemes were costly because of the need to provide cover for the GP and because of the staff resource they require. One-to-one mentoring and peer support were also common across the LIZ. Because of the intensity of the relationship, mentoring was felt to be particularly susceptible to conflicting agendas. Conditions for success included: clear identification, perhaps in the form of a written agreement, of objectives and a specification of expectations; proper records and structured feedback; and regular meetings of mentors in order to provide them with support.

GPs' self-directed learning strategies: 'big bidders' and 'accumulators'

Madeleine Gantley, Jo Tissier, Alex Jamieson, Tony Rennison and Maggie Aiken

In East London, the evaluation of GPs' use of LIZEI funding was conducted jointly by the Department of General Practice and Primary Care of St Bartholomew's and the Royal London School of Medicine and Dentistry, and Thames Postgraduate Medical and Dental Education. By the end of LIZEI our database held 2,648 records of educational activities by the 360 GPs in Hackney, Newham and Tower Hamlets. This allowed us to look at uptake by individual GPs and by practice, and by a range of different GP and practice parameters. The database provided a broad summary of activities, the characteristics of those who claimed and those who did not, and allowed us to identify different patterns of claims for LIZEI funding. Four different patterns of use of LIZEI funding were identified:

- academic trainees
- big bidders
- accumulators
- non-bidders.

Academic trainees (AT) encompass both LATS (London Academic Trainee Scheme) and academic fellows. They are young GPs who have completed their vocational training schemes, the former doing three sessions a week in practices, and the latter five sessions a week. The aim was both to provide these young GPs with academic training, and to provide help to practices in an area in which recruitment of new GPs is difficult, and locums rarely available.

Academic trainees came into the LIZEI scheme either through responding to advertisements in the medical media, or through membership of local information networks. Their principal motivation lay in the potential of the scheme to provide them with 'breathing space' at a time when their personal and professional lives were uncertain.

'I wasn't sure what I wanted and where I wanted to be and in my personal life at the time … long term, and so I didn't want to commit myself to a partnership at that stage'.

The evaluation revealed some conflict between the AT priorities (to improve their academic skills and to develop their clinical skills) and those of the practice (long-term help with heavy clinical workload). While ATs found support within the department of general practice for improving academic skills, there appeared to be a lack of provision for clinical support, a lack of clarity about whether the Department or the host practice should be providing this, and a two-way lack of understanding about the 'other half' of the AT role.

The second most evident mode of involvement we have termed the **'big bidders'**. These were typically GPs who had early knowledge of the availability of funds, either individual GPs who received large sums of money for one-off activities such as doing an MSc or writing a book, or groups of GPs within a practice who submitted co-ordinated bids. GPs adopted both proactive and reactive strategies:

- proactive being the use of the funds for an activity they wished to undertake anyway, such as a master's degree:

  'My approach to LIZEI was entirely instrumental'.

- reactive being essentially responsive to the range of courses available which was widely seen as allowing GPs more flexibility than the PGEA agenda:

  'The course just caught my eye for some reason'.

For some GPs, motivation changed with their involvement in longer courses. The GP cited above as adopting a reactive learning strategy described having no clear educational objectives at the start of a course, but on completion realising that the process had prompted a renewed interest in his own learning:

'I'm not in the same position now that I was two years ago, where I only did it because I was going to get paid for it'.

The drawbacks identified by these GPs lay first in the political domain, with some GPs having a clear view that the funding was a political sweetener for GPs in London, particularly following the Tomlinson reforms. In addition, their ability to make use of the funding was limited by the lack of availability of locums. Concerns were raised about equity in allocation: were they being made available simply to those who were already relatively well-placed, relatively well-funded practices, and politically adept GPs? Why was the funding available only to GPs and not to other members of the primary health care team?

The **accumulators** had different ways of accessing the LIZEI money. They spoke of confusion about both the availability of funds, and how to access them. In addition, they had no clear ideas about what their educational needs were, or how to identify them. This meant that they were 'late starters', and needed help in the practice to get them off the ground. (The database shows a pattern of claiming in years two and three, and more claims from GPs in fundholding or multifund practices, and more from older GPs – the 49–59 year age group.) The most valuable source of help these GPs found was in the provision of long-term assistants through LIZEI, via a series of grants rather than a one-off scheme such as that of the ATs:

'Without an assistant in place, I don't think either of us would have had the inclination or time to think or to develop these services'.

The 'accumulators' also spoke of the value of peer support which emerged as they started to become involved in educational activities, some of them for the first time in many years of practice:

'Because of LIZEI this group started, and if there was no LIZEI, it would possibly never have started … The doctors who are 45–65 are the main group who participated'

'It made me realise that we can do our own education'

GPs also described the realisation that they could take charge of their own education, and establish their own locally relevant agenda, rather than follow the traditional postgraduate education model. The innovative style of learning developed in the self-directed learning groups has continued beyond the period of LIZEI funding.

GPs recognised the value of the opportunity to compare their own knowledge and skills with those of their colleagues, a particularly important aspect for single-handed practitioners:

> *'To find out how I compare with other doctors [on the same course] – this in small practices you can't find out'.*

On the other hand, they identified tensions between their practice commitments and the educational activities they wished to undertake; again they spoke of inequity and randomness in the way funding was allocated, and the short-term nature of the funding.

Finally, the **non-bidders**, while difficult both to contact and to interview, identified a lack of time and information, and giving priority to their heavy clinical workload. For some there was active hostility to the whole LIZEI enterprise, which was seen as inequitable, with a lack of focus on those GPs who stood to benefit most; for others the concern was with the essentially short-term nature of the project.

In summary, the key influences affecting GPs' use of LIZEI funds were:

- access to information (on availability of funds, educational courses or help services such as facilitation)
- equity in allocation of funds, both among GPs and among members of the primary health care team
- a variety of educational activities to meet the needs of different learning styles
- the stage of individual professional and educational development
- the stage of practice development.

While those GPs with proactive learning strategies clearly achieved their own individual learning needs, perhaps the most notable aspect of the contribution of LIZEI to GP education lies among those whose strategy was essentially reactive, taking shorter or longer courses or joining learning groups. The evidence from the self-directed learning groups, in terms of both GPs setting their own educational agenda and the opportunity for calibration of knowledge and skills with peers, suggests real evidence of the educational 'refreshment' of GPs that was one of the initial aims of LIZEI.

Learning from the LIZEI

These two contributions portray LIZEI as a gigantic natural experiment in new forms of continuing professional development for GPs. The scale of the experiment, and the enormous diversity of activities it encompassed made evaluation particularly complex. Nevertheless, a number of lessons can be identified:

- LIZEI money came on stream with insufficient notice, and the programme would have benefited from a one- or two-year planning period
- educational boards of all stakeholders have been beneficial in breaking down boundaries between partners, and co-ordinating activity across the education/service divide
- An approach which focused on the practice as well as the individual members of the team benefited team building, and service delivery
- the role of health authorities needed to be carefully negotiated, particularly as they also have a monitoring role
- active involvement of HAs can ensure that patient and population needs stay on the agenda
- addressing the professional development needs of GP principals in isolation compromises the notion of the multiprofessional primary health care team
- GPs adopted different but recognisable approaches to the use of LIZEI funding that reflected different learning styles, their level of educational and practice development
- there are large numbers of non-principal GPs working in London whose needs have not been addressed by the programme (although some boards did try to target non-principals)

- practice visits were a valuable part of the educational development, and can have additional benefits. However, if GPs see them as monitoring their performance they will be unlikely to participate
- the protected time funded through the LIZEI was seen as a major factor in promoting high take-up
- providing protected time is expensive; over half the education board budget has been spent on this
- three years are insufficient to achieve radical change in GPs learning habits, and many may revert to the traditional PGEA approach to CPD
- considerable expertise has been developed in London as a result of the programme, but with the end of special funding this resource could be dissipated.

References

Department of Health (1993). *Making London Better (The Tomlinson Report)*. London: HMSO

LIZEI Annual Report 1996/97. London: NHS Executive North Thames & South Thames

LIZ GP Incentives Project Team (1998). *Proceedings of the workshop on continuing professional development for established GPs funded under LIZEI*. December 1997. GP Research Paper

Chapter 4

General practice as a learning environment

Alison Hill and Geoffrey Norris

KEY POINTS

- Continuing education must be relevant, engaging and flexible

- In an ideal learning organisation all members are both teachers and learners

- Because of the demands of a busy practice, learning activity there must be carefully planned and managed

- Learning should be directed towards shared goals, while respecting the needs and perspectives of the individual

- A practice-based learning environment must be nurtured through open communication and explicit team objectives

This chapter explores the need for continuing education for the practice team, the extent to which continuing education can be based in the workplace, and the opportunities and challenges this will present.

Continuing professional development and NHS policy

Increasingly, primary health care is seen as the business of teams of generalists drawn from different professions. These bring their differing perspectives and skills to bear on the patient-centred delivery of integrated programmes or packages of care. However, this idea challenges general practices as primary care providers for two reasons. First, the degree of organisational sophistication is insufficiently advanced. The development of individuals needs to be integrated with current thinking about continuing professional education, and about evidence-based practice in its broadest sense. Professional morale needs to be improved through appropriate support and continuing training. Second, diverse groups seldom come together already equipped to play a full part in the team. Working successfully together implies learning together and from each other.

Continuing professional development in practice

Most of the research evidence about the effectiveness of educating adults is based on work with middle-class white Americans, and should therefore be applied with caution to the needs of those working in primary care in the NHS.

Adults do not have to learn actively: it is not their first priority when they are engaged in practice. Continuing education therefore must be relevant and engaging, and it must meet their needs: there must be something in it for them, and it must take account of their maturity. However much individuals are altruistically committed to caring for patients and to promoting good relationships with colleagues, learning must first hold the promise of personal growth before it can be expected to benefit patients; and must meet the individuals' professional accreditation requirements before it can benefit the organisation as a whole.

There is much to be gained from adults learning in groups but educational provision needs to be flexible. For example, some people like to learn by experimentation, others like to research a topic from libraries, or attend a formal course or perhaps watch an expert. Not only may individuals have differing preferences in the way they learn best, they may also have different levels of knowledge or of academic attainment. Teaching and learning in mixed groups can therefore be particularly challenging.

There is at present much interest in teaching and learning in the practice. The expectations are, first, that the commitment to find the time might be enhanced if travel to an outside location is avoided, and if many or all of the staff are involved. Second, such an inclusive approach should contribute to the development of a team's identity and common purpose.

Learning for individuals and for organisations

There is an increasing recognition that for organisations to develop they must attend to those learning needs of the individuals that are relevant to their role in the organisation. Learning from commercial practice, the NHS sees staff development as a key responsibility. The recently published report of the CMO's Working Party (1998) on continuing professional development in general practice recommends that the focus of activity should be development plans for individual practices, aimed at meeting the needs of their patients and of the NHS. The concept of the Practice Professional Development Plan recognises the whole practice as a human resource for health care in proposing an integrated programme of professional development for the practice team. This is an ambitious idea and assumes that if individuals work with a common purpose they can benefit from learning together.

Such proposals avoid the questions related to the relative efficacy of multidisciplinary, multiprofessional and interprofessional education. Multidisciplinary learning implies that education is not the sole preserve of a single profession or discipline. Teachers and learners may come from different professional backgrounds. The key skill for the teacher is the facilitation of learning. Interprofessional education implies that members of different professions learn from each other in a co-operative and egalitarian way that is grounded in practice and derived from experience. Ideally, multidisciplinary learning should involve a similar exchange, although the assumption is that the learners as a group are motivated by a wish to benefit from the teacher's knowledge. Ideally, also, in multiprofessional settings, all participants should learn from each other.

When members of a practice learn together, it is likely to be in the interprofessional mode, but individuals may have to work hard to break down boundaries related to historical training patterns, and learn to acknowledge the expertise of others, as well as their differing perspectives and needs. GPs and nurses, for example, have differing professional expectations in terms of their continued training and accreditation which may affect the individuals' priorities for learning.

With the increasing emphasis on the integration of different professionals in primary care teams and in the proposed PCGs, it seems sensible for teams to learn together and from each other. It could be convenient, relevant, interactive, engaging, focused on patient care, and collaborative. But the leap from recommendations to reality has to bridge many practical and attitudinal difficulties.

The practice as a place of learning

The advantages of practice-based learning relate to its relevance to the work of the practice and its members. In particular, it should emphasise the interplay between the various roles of individuals. Although the practice is a relatively small organisation, it can capitalise on the large body of knowledge and the wide range of experience and perspectives to be found within it. However, finding the time and using opportunities for learning most effectively, towards relevant and agreed goals, will need planning, management and leadership.

There are real weaknesses in educational terms in a workplace approach to education. Within practices there are hierarchies. These are dominated by doctors. They are the employers of many of the other members of the team and the paternalistic nature of their training and professionalisation leads them to expect to be the leaders in any group. Gender differences may exacerbate hierarchical differences, as may variation in formal educational attainment. In addition, there may be differing views of the value or relevance of any educational activity, and it may be difficult to persuade everyone to take the time out of practice. In LIZEI the cardinal feature was that funding was available to pay for GPs' time, allowing many doctors in small practices to employ locums and assistants.

One advantage of learning which takes place outside the practice is that participants from other groups may bring new ideas and fresh perspectives.

Self-directed learning

It is widely believed that the most effective learning for adults is self-directed. It implies independence and an understanding of personal learning need. It is important that a sense of autonomy is preserved to minimise feelings of coercion and threat since such feelings and the associated anxiety are likely to reduce the quality of any learning that might take place.

One of the most exciting developments funded by LIZEI has been self-directed learning groups. These have been uniprofessional and represent the first stage in breaking down the barriers to learning together in a collaborative and non-threatening way. Many participants had not experienced participative education before, and found it empowering and refreshing. The groups themselves have in some cases been led by GPs who had not been involved formally in the delivery or management of education. With relatively little training they have been able to take on this role and have emerged as charismatic leaders of their peers.

However, there is a suspicion that if left to themselves, individuals will not stray outside their 'comfort zone', tend not to address difficult areas and learn what they really need to know. Evidence from CME in Canada has demonstrated that clinicians, if left to learn only what they choose, concentrate on what they already know, to the detriment of improving their knowledge in their weaker areas (Sibley et al. 1982). Co-tutoring has helped this problem, as have schemes using educational mentors.

It is likely that any programme of self-directed learning will have the goals of increased competence and enhanced performance. These are equally likely to be the expectations of NHS management and employers. Indeed, the goals of education for learners are both self-centred and related to social role. Health professionals have both the right to the realisation of their potential and a duty to equip themselves to do what society expects. These expectations are explicit when set out in professional standards and regulations, and implicit in widely held cultural beliefs and morality. The learners' needs then will be directed towards the attainment of these goals. However, besides this emphasis on self-directed learning, external views of the skill and knowledge deficits related to the needs of the service must also be taken into account. For example, if the local prescribing figures for inhaled asthma treatment suggest that practices are not following accepted treatment guidelines, education should support more rational prescribing, even if the doctors themselves do not see this as a priority.

When the organisation as a whole is considered, the picture becomes more complex. Three sets of learning needs may be identified, although there will be overlap between them:

- the needs of the team in order to perform the task
- the needs of the individuals within the team to allow them to play fully their particular roles
- the needs of the group to maintain itself as a working group.

Learning by reflecting on practice

Much learning in adult life is based on practice, and expertise is gained through experience. Much of this learning is unconscious. However, the learning is more enjoyable and more effective if the analysis of the experience of practice, and particularly of unusual incidents, is undertaken in a supportive way. New experiences are then put into the context of individual knowledge, tested against the benchmark of current knowledge and then internalised as new knowledge. This process has been called reflective practice, and its use in educating professionals described by Donald Schön in his classic text (Schön 1988).

Schön argues that through developing the skills of learning in action, professionals are better equipped to continue learning throughout their professional lives, and to use a changing knowledge base to solve problems that do not fit precisely into established theory. For practical problems rarely do. Reflective practice leads to sustained learning, and sustainable changes in practice for the better. Using such an approach to the development of practice based on evidence, when so little research evidence is as yet derived from primary health care, promises to be helpful.

There seems to be a logical progression from applying this approach to the education of individuals to that of groups such as a practice team: the practice becomes a learning organism.

Service and education: is there a tension?

Learning in the practice needs to promote the ability of the team and its individual members to meet the needs of patients in the most efficient, effective and humane way possible. Concern is often expressed that when NHS management and employers talk about the education and training agenda for those who deliver the care, they are seeking to impose a pattern of learning unsympathetic to the needs of the professionals and at odds with their values.

Conflicting priorities

There may be a conflict between the interests of the individual practice in terms of its overarching purpose, and the obligations of outside agencies such as health authorities, who rely on provider organisations such as practices to deliver patient care. How a practice prioritises its activities may therefore be different from the view held by outside agencies. For example, a health authority, conscious of its poor performance on *Health of the Nation* targets and the morbidity patterns of its population may wish the practice to develop its service to diabetic patients, or its child health promotion programme. The practice, on the other hand, sees little income or interest in taking full responsibility for its diabetic patients, when there is a convenient service offered at the local hospital, whereas it is keen to develop a new andrology service, using new techniques available to primary care through new therapeutic products. The health authority is concerned about the cost of those products and sees no need for services additional to those provided by the local urino-genitary specialists.

The need to negotiate

These tensions can be managed, provided a dialogue is established between outside agencies and the practices. This needs to recognise leadership issues, change management and negotiating skills. Respect for the other's perspective and priorities is just as important in this setting as it is in developing a learning organisation within the practice. Once ways have been found to manage these tensions, agreement on the prioritisation of educational activity towards shared goals should follow. One of the most pervading tensions may be between the health authority's view of service need and the educational effort required to meet new contractual requirements. The financial reward for new service contracts will need to be commensurate with the learning effort involved.

The way forward

In summary, in an ideal learning organisation, all members are both teachers and learners. Learning is planned and is directed towards shared goals while respecting the needs and perspectives of individuals. The whole organisation shares the desire to provide high-quality care in an environment that is free from blame, coercion and exploitation. Learning without a purpose is not merely self-indulgent, but is likely to be ineffective and a waste of time. Active learning requires the ability to question accepted practice, a spirit of enquiry and the tools to access information and knowledge from both within the organisation and outside it. Learning with people from other professions and from across hierarchical boundaries requires motivation, understanding and courage.

Although the practice as a learning organisation is devoted to progress, its main purpose is to treat patients. Primary care being the first point of access to health care, general practice work can be unpredictable and its demands heavy. Learning activity will therefore have to be carefully planned and managed. Several models have been proposed, variously focusing on process and outcome (Al-Sheri *et al.* 1993).

It would be unrealistic to suggest that continuing professional development in primary care will be entirely served by an interprofessional, practice-based approach. However, the main advantage of mutual learning in the workplace is that new knowledge can be put into practice straightaway, with the support of those who have shared in that learning, whereas when new knowledge is brought in from outside the practice, there is often a complex process of negotiation, learning and acceptance to be gone through, before effective and sustainable change occurs in the practice. Not all learning can be internally resourced, and there will be a need for expert educational support, facilitation, or technical expertise, from outside.

Learning contracts for practices?

The CMO's working group suggests a strategic approach, with the practice's professional development plan based on its business development plan. Experience with individual CPD shows that it takes considerable time and independent mentorship or advice to produce a coherent and manageable personal learning plan. How long it will take a practice team to learn how to produce effective staff development and practice learning plans can only be imagined.

In order to encourage such a developmental step, contracts for educational activity may need to be considered.

Stakeholders in the learning contract

The practice plans will have to take into account local and district-wide health need, will have to fit in with the strategic frameworks provided by local PCGs and by educational consortia, and with the health authority's health improvement programme. They should address the issue of where the balance of responsibility for such education will lie, and the matter of the source and level of funding dedicated to staff development (DoH 1996, 1997).

Resourcing the plans

Practices will need to be adept at accessing external expertise and advice in producing their plans and in delivering their education. Partnerships with other professions, such as community pharmacy, might be useful, as might expertise from health authorities, academic institutions and independent training organisations, as well as the traditional sources from the hospital sector. Increasingly, voluntary organisations and medical charities are keen to be involved in the education and training of health professionals.

Practices will need a budget to pay for this activity. Currently, funding for education in primary care comes through the MADEL budget, GMS cash-limited payments, health service trust and the pharmaceutical industry. Soon, the funding of education of non-medical primary care staff will be managed by local education consortia. But at present, taking advantage of funding opportunities requires a creative approach that is often stifled by NHS regulations, which in some cases preclude all members of the team benefiting from certain types of funding. A budget will need to be in place before learning contracts for practices can become a reality, although that would not preclude practices using several sources of funding to support their educational programmes. With the current government policy emphasis on lifelong learning, funding may be available from outside the health arena.

Educational and political imperatives

The learning environment of the practice will in many cases need to be nurtured. Those responsible at all levels for both the professional and organisational development of primary care must actively encourage a range of features within practices, ranging from skilled leadership and a 'no-blame' culture, to open communication and explicit team objectives. PCGs will not soon supplant practices as a focus for these activities and must take care not to undermine them.

The proposals of the CMO's working party and the intentions expressed in the Government's White Paper must be implemented with respect and understanding for the purpose, tasks and priorities of primary care professionals as learners. They must be adequately supported and funded. The educational plans must have clear objectives and should be properly evaluated both internally and by those responsible for ensuring the efficiency and effectiveness of the NHS as a whole. Then primary care practitioners could take responsibility for the continued identification and satisfaction of their learning needs: truly continuing professional education in the practice as a learning environment.

References

Al-Sheri A, Stanley I, Thomas P (1993). Continuing education for general practice. 2. Systematic learning from experience. *BJGP* 43:249–53

Chief Medical Officer (1998). *A review of continuing professional development in general practice*. London: HMSO

Department of Health (1996). *A service with ambitions*. London: The Stationery Office

Department of Health (1997). *The new NHS*. London: The Stationery Office

Schön DA (1988). *Educating the reflective practitioner towards a new design for teaching and learning in the professions*. San Francisco (CA): Basic Books Inc.

Sibley JC, Sackett DC, Neufield V *et al.* (1982). A randomised trial of continuing medical education. *New England Journal of Medicine* 306:511–15

Chapter 5

The impact of the education–service partnership on service quality

Trisha Greenhalgh and John Eversley

KEY POINTS

- The challenge to develop valid measures of quality in general practice has attracted interest from a wide range of professional and lay groups.

- While efforts to define measures of structure, process and outcome in primary care have met with some success, the core features of general practice remain difficult to define and even more difficult to measure.

- The notion of a unitary, one-dimensional index that can be used for the assessment of all aspects of quality in general practice is a dangerous illusion. Different groups should recognise that their different objectives necessarily require different measures of quality.

Why does anybody care about education for GPs? Contributions elsewhere in this book show that there are a variety of reasons. Education is paid for by the Government as a means of improving quality. The 'four Rs' were discussed in Chapter 2: recruitment, retention, reflection and refreshment. Two more Rs, regulation and reward, might also be added. Earlier contributions emphasise the role of education in promoting high-quality health care. The individual GP's motivation in taking part varies enormously, as demonstrated by Judy Gilley from the GMSC (now GPC) and in Chapter 3 reviewing the LIZEI programme. However, for many GPs, personal and professional development is also about quality. As many contributors to this volume indicate, education is increasingly judged by participants' capability, or what they achieve as a result of taking part in a programme. Education then is to be judged, in part, by its impact on quality. For all these reasons, knowing what we mean by 'quality' is crucial.

The vision

It is widely believed that the increasing involvement of primary care teams in undergraduate education will improve standards. In attempting to meet criteria for becoming a teaching practice, GPs will update their practice libraries, improve the standard of record-keeping, go on courses, and work towards postgraduate qualifications. Training of GP tutors by specialists will refresh their clinical skills, update them on developments in particular specialties and encourage the use of evidence-based protocols for diagnosis, treatment and referral.

The presence of inquisitive students in the practice will spur GPs to do their job thoroughly, reflect on different aspects of their practice, and look up information in textbooks and journals. Dedicated funding will allow purchase of both teaching and clinical equipment. GPs, previously the most professionally isolated of doctors, will be connected to hospitals, libraries, academic departments of primary care and the Internet, via state-of-the-art computer systems.

Of course, this optimistic vision fails to address a number of important issues in the debate. Both the definition and the measurement of quality in primary care are highly controversial areas. Standards of care do not automatically rise when new objectives are set, and a new infrastructure is created. Financial rewards for teaching students could potentially act as perverse incentives and attract conscripts, rather than partners, to the scheme. Enthusiasm for teaching, and the novelty of the initiative, could divert time and resources away from patient care. Practice staff who find themselves bearing an additional service burden while the enthusiasts spend more time in the classroom may become resentful, with knock-on effects on practice dynamics. Patients who previously valued a continuing and intimate relationship with their family doctor may find that relationship subtly disturbed by the intermittent presence of successive cohorts of students.

Principles of quality indicators

The task of developing quality indicators begs the question 'what will those indicators be used for?', and immediately raises important political issues. Such indicators, for example, may serve as:

- a focus for individual GPs, or groups of GPs, to reflect on their own practice and plan their professional development
- a framework for describing the current status of general practice at a district, regional, or national level
- a means of assessing whether particular policy interventions such as LIZEI have been effective in raising standards
- a tool for measuring (and, implicitly, penalising or rewarding) the performance of individual GPs or practices, and recording improvement or deterioration over time
- a means of defining standards and identifying individuals, practices or health authorities who fail to meet them, i.e. a means of accountability (upwards) and performance management (downwards)
- a way of informing or justifying the allocation of limited resources to practices
- a source of information for service users.

No indicators can exist in a social, cultural or political vacuum. Quality indicators may be 'objective' in that what they measure can be expressed quantitatively and shown to be reproducible. But the temptation to see such indicators as a unitary, all-encompassing reflection of external truth, should be strongly resisted.

Although there is currently some debate in health management circles about the precise definition of primary care, and in professional circles about the current and future role of the GP, we have taken the pragmatic view that primary care is what primary care practitioners currently do. Good primary care is good at being itself – i.e. at being accessible, ongoing, comprehensive and co-ordinated front-line care that improves well-being, extends life expectancy and keeps people out of hospital where appropriate.

It has been customary to group quality indicators under the following headings:

- **Structure** – includes size and state of repair of premises, disabled access, presence of a treatment room, computerisation, patient-to-staff ratio, presence of equipment (autoclave, ECG machine, minor surgery equipment, etc.), languages spoken in the surgery

- **Process** – includes waiting times, consultation length, rate of uptake of services (e.g. cervical smear rates), patient satisfaction, rates of health-damaging behaviours (e.g. smoking), equity of access to services (e.g. across different minority ethnic groups)

- **Outcome** – covers levels of physical, psychological or social health status, quality of life, equity in health status (e.g. across different socio-economic groups).

This classification should not, however, be applied too rigidly in the context of general practice. For example, as we argue below, 'patient satisfaction' in primary care is closely related to what Howie *et al.* (1991) have described as 'enablement', a variable that might be viewed as an outcome in itself. Whereas in commercial sectors the 'customer care' aspects of quality are often readily separable from the product itself, the same cannot be said of quality in primary care. Furthermore, the above classification focuses exclusively on the measurable, perhaps at the expense of an initial philosophical reflection on what exactly we mean by quality in general practice. For these reasons, we have avoided the structure-process-outcome classification.

Other headings for quality indicators, which we discuss in more detail below, include the following:

- measures of the 'good consultation', 'good doctor', or 'good practice' derived either from patients' declared values or from a theoretical perspective
- targets and performance indicators (usually derived from the structure-process-outcome schema)
- professional standards for education and training (and entry criteria derived from these)
- aspects of clinical or organisational audit
- practice of evidence-based medicine (often wrongly equated with adherence to guidelines)
- organisational behaviour of the primary health care team.

However quality is defined, the indicator(s) chosen to measure it should ideally be:

- reliable
- reproducible
- easily quantifiable (using readily available information)
- affordable.

If the level of the indicator changes that should indicate better or worse quality depending on whether it increases or decreases. Indicators should also measure a useful, important and relevant aspect of care. They should be true predictors of quality. Each should be both sensitive, i.e. a high score on the indicator should indicate quality in a particular aspect of care, and specific, so that a low score should indicate that the quality of this aspect of care is inadequate. They should be amenable to quality-control monitoring designed to distinguish cosmetic changes from genuine improvements.

It should be possible to use the data they provide to produce comparative and aggregated data between and across practices. Changes in the levels of quality indicators should rapidly and accurately reflect the success of attempts to improve the quality of care.

Quality in primary care: whose perspective?

Those who define quality from within a single discipline or role tend to have little difficulty reaching consensus with their colleagues on what counts as good, mediocre or poor performance. Indeed, there is remarkable agreement *within* different professional, administrative and lay groups on the principles for measuring quality in general practice.

Difficulties occur when the different groups come together and find that each has built their definition of quality, and proposed system of evaluation, around a different set of underlying values and priorities.

Although in recent years there has rightly been increasing emphasis on the 'evidence-based' management of patients in primary care, the 1990s have also seen a resurgence of the subjective aspects, or what some have dubbed the 'human side', of general practice (Evan & Sweeney 1998).

It is well recognised that the empathic, listening, witness-bearing aspect of care is difficult to define and difficult to measure. How, asks Pereira Gray (1992), does one decide whether a generalist doctor relating to a 'whole person' has or has not made an impact, has or has not done a good job, and whether or not the patient is any better? Given that the sharing of the patient's illness experience is also a uniquely private event that may not be consciously recognised by patient or doctor, nor recorded systematically in case notes, it is small wonder that this aspect is all too easily ignored when constructing a set of competencies for the modern GP.

It is important for any set of quality standards to reflect, in addition to measures of where and how general practice interfaces with secondary care, the essence of general practice itself.

Measuring the quality of my consultations

The consultation is the core unit of general practice. In the eyes of most patients, the chief role of the family doctor is for patient-initiated consultations. Some years ago it was shown that for patients the three most important features of a good GP were 'doctor listens to me', 'doctor sorts out my problems' and 'I usually see the same doctor' (Smith & Armstrong 1989).

In a series of preliminary observational studies on GPs, and using each GP as his or her own control, Professor John Howie and colleagues in Edinburgh defined higher quality care as occurring when more attention was given to physical and psychosocial elements, when preventive care was offered, when less medication was prescribed for trivial illness, and when patients expressed greater satisfaction with the consultation. They demonstrated that, thus defined, quality of care was inversely related to the doctor's own perception of stress, and also directly related to consultation length. They showed that longer consultations (those lasting ten minutes or more) were associated with more specific benefits to patients compared with short ones (lasting five minutes or less), and offered the long-to-short consultation ratio as a proxy measure of quality in the consultation (Howie *et al.* 1991).

In a subsequent study, the same authors grouped doctors into 'more' or 'less' patient-centred, and showed that doctors who were most stressed combined a patient-centred consulting style (which tended to be slower) with either overbooked surgeries or poor time management, so that they regularly ran late and felt that they had short-changed their patients.

Howie and colleagues then developed and validated a number of more definitive instruments for the measurement of quality in the consultation. At the individual level, longer consulting time was generally associated with greater enablement (i.e. greater satisfaction and greater ability to cope with the illness and life in general). Practices who allocated more time for consulting generally had higher levels of enablement in their patients. Furthermore, at doctor level, those who spent longer with their patients produced more enablement than 'faster' consulters. Given that this was an observational study, it must be remembered that subtle differences in case mix may explain part or all of the variation between doctors, even though case mix as measured by the needs questionnaire did not differ between doctors.

Howie and colleagues have shown that their 'enablement' questionnaire is reliable and is valid for the Scottish population used in their studies so far. They plan to compare it with other satisfaction questionnaires developed in secondary care, and also to pilot the instrument in different minority ethnic groups. In an ongoing validation project, the social aspects of the needs questionnaire may also be compared with deprivation indices such as the Jarman index. The authors are enthusiastic about the potential for the 'enablement' instrument to provide a marker for holistic care in general practice.

The 'activity' perspective: performance indicators and targets

Health authorities, which have a statutory duty to monitor the quality of GPs' performance and limited resources for achieving this task, generally try to assess quality by means of routinely collected data such as levels of immunisation or cervical smear uptake, or the nature and cost of prescribed drugs. Indeed, the use of routinely collected and regularly updated quantitative data as quality indicators has so much intuitive appeal from the purchaser's perspective that some may fail to question the validity, reliability or comprehensiveness of measures.

The stance generally taken by health authorities defines general practice as a set of activities, which Bosanquet (1995) has classified into:

- demand-led consultations
- disease management
- screening and risk factor assessment
- referral to/organising secondary care.

In a report entitled *Defining Core Services*, the General Medical Services Committee of the British Medical Association has suggested a similar classification as a basis for financial negotiations between GPs and health authorities:

Category A: services normally provided by GPs when responding to perceived need

Category B: proactive care such as health promotion or new patient medicals

Category C: practice services commonly provided but not included in core Category A, such as immunisations, child health surveillance, cervical cytology, and monitoring of diabetes and asthma

Category D: additional services provided by GPs with specialist training (e.g. minor surgery, intrapartum care)

Category E: organisation of care (e.g. administration of out of hours, screening programmes, etc.)

Category F: recruitment and organisation of practice staff.

The most notable feature of the GMSC report is that it explicitly avoids offering an all-encompassing definition of 'the services normally provided by every GP when responding to patients' (Category A services above). Much of the document, and indeed much of the literature on so-called quality indicators in general practice as well as virtually all specific performance targets for practice-based activity so far introduced at health authority level, concern additional services such as those in Categories B to F above.

In the light of the above discussion about the patient's perspective, performance indicators constructed from items in these supplementary categories should be viewed, at best, as measuring a small part of what goes on in primary care.

Targets

The 1990 GP contract set specific targets for certain operational goals in primary care, and linked GP incomes to achievement of these goals. The national health strategies (*The Health of the Nation, Our Healthier Nation*) have also taken a target-setting approach. The research literature on target setting in primary care has been reviewed by Elkin and Robinson (1997) who conclude that targets have a number of drawbacks as quality indicators:

- targets focus on things that are easily measured
- they may be unrealistic or even unattainable in certain population groups
- they may foster complacency among those who have already achieved the upper target level
- targets may act as a disincentive, since those who perceive even the lower target level as unattainable may abandon all activity in that area
- national targets may skew local priorities
- they may fail to reflect the variation in needs, access to health services or willingness to accept services between different practice populations
- targets may widen inequalities in health, since efforts may be directed not at those most in need but rather at those most likely to accept the services offered
- achievement of targets may not be associated with better patient-relevant outcomes
- targets can be manipulated, sometimes to the detriment of patient care (e.g. meeting a target for childhood immunisations by removing all children who are not immunised from the list)
- the opportunity cost of efforts to achieve targets (i.e. the effect on health gain in other areas) should be assessed as well as performance

against the target itself; even when change is achieved, efforts and resources might be better spent elsewhere.

Targets as currently constructed tend to reflect the priorities of doctors (i.e. crude measures of illness levels and premature death) rather than nurses (i.e. symptom control, psychological health, and quality of life).

In addition, the concept of targets as conceived, for example, in the 1990 GP contract, is predicated upon a 'medical' view of illness which conspicuously neglects the social determinants of ill health, such as poverty, unemployment and poor housing. Thus, the health needs of isolated, housebound elderly people are defined as being partially met by an annual visit from the GP rather than by an increase in state pensions or fuel subsidies.

Nevertheless, there is evidence that target setting for particular aspects of care has been successful in changing practice and achieving health gain, most notably in the field of cervical cytology. However, the gap between 'leading edge' and 'trailing edge' practices in this area shows no sign of narrowing, and coverage of minority ethnic groups remains inadequate, partly for administrative rather than cultural reasons.

The 'gatekeeper' perspective: investigation, admission and referral rates

In health care, more is not always better. Much of the illness (and perceived illness) seen in primary care is self-limiting. It is often good practice to dissuade patients from having the blood test, X-ray or specialist opinion they seek. Referral rates for cataract removal, tonsillectomy, and uterine dilatation and curettage have all been cited as suitable markers of the 'gatekeeping' function of the GP. But low referral rates are not always a sign of excellence, since the assiduous search for unmet need almost always uncovers conditions that require secondary care input.

It cannot be assumed that GPs refer patients to specialists either for assessment or treatment of a condition that unequivocally needs specialist management, or, alternatively, to avoid doing the work themselves. More usually, referral occurs for a complex set of reasons which include uncertainty about diagnosis, concern about length of waiting lists, inadequate information exchange between primary and secondary care, and inability to access certain investigations without an initial outpatient consultation. The situation is made more complex by the fact that GPs' referral data are not universally available, and hospital activity statistics are usually used as a proxy. It is highly debatable whether the appropriateness of referrals can ever be determined on the basis of hospital outpatient activity rates or finished consultant episodes. Random variation in morbidity might explain much of the variability between practices.

There are, however, some specific aspects of contact with secondary care which could potentially be validated as marker conditions for inappropriate primary care. There is limited evidence, for example, that acute admission rates for asthma are a reliable reflection of the adequacy of a practice's asthma service (British Thoracic Society 1997), and the same can probably be said of the so-called neglect-related complications of diabetes (foot ulceration, sight-threatening retinopathy, and acute metabolic decompensation). Other conditions for which avoidable admissions have been used as quality indicators are epilepsy, acute heart failure, urinary tract infection and gastro-enteritis. However, such dramatic events are relatively rare even in patients receiving inadequate care, and incidence figures will be easily skewed by a single atypical case, so they are, at best, a crude measure of quality, especially in small practices.

The economic perspective: effective and cost-effective prescribing

Medication, like investigation or referral, is often not strictly necessary, and some researchers have used high prescribing rates in themselves as an indicator of quality. This general principle is, however, more valid in some prescribing situations than others. Whereas a high rate of cephalosporin prescribing for acute respiratory illness in a general practice population is not justifiable on rational grounds, there is good evidence to support the claim that a low rate of prescribing of inhaled steroids (and other preventive medication) compared to bronchodilators indicates poor asthma care, and that underprescription of drugs such as aspirin and warfarin contributes to avoidable strokes in high risk patients. Once again, the active search for unmet need in conditions such as diabetes and hypertension will increase costs.

Lipid-lowering treatment, especially with statin drugs, is expensive but, in the long term, cost-effective in carefully defined groups of patients. Where resources are limited, therefore, high crude rates of statin prescribing cannot be equated with either good or poor quality care.

Different individuals, and different subgroups within a practice population, have different needs (and different expectations) for prescribed medication. The question of whether it is possible to derive a mathematical formula that successfully predicts legitimate variation in prescribing costs between practices and exposes (with a view to penalising) idiosyncratic variation is a controversial subject (Greenhalgh 1998, Majeed & Head 1998). Adjustment for demographic variables, socioeconomic status and standardised illness indicators accounts for only a minority of the variation in prescribing costs between practices. But these same variables account for 81 per cent of the variation in net ingredient cost between patients at health authority level, suggesting that factors other than illness rates and sociodemographic factors explain most of the variability in prescribing costs between individual GPs.

The total prescribing costs of a GP practice will be determined by a complex interplay of factors that militates against the computation of a unitary, one-dimensional index of prescribing quality. Particular aspects of prescribing have been identified by the Audit Commission (1994) as explaining a high proportion of idiosyncratic variation in GP prescribing. According to their report, if the worst-performing practices were brought up to the level of the best, considerable savings could be made at no detriment (and some benefit) to patient care. The four aspects of prescribing defined by the Audit Commission as valid indicators of quality in GP prescribing are:

- generic prescribing rate
- use of a preferred list of drugs (formulary) to ensure that the most

effective and cost-effective medication is selected for a particular condition

- rate of prescribing of drugs identified as having limited therapeutic efficacy (e.g. appetite suppressants) or having cheaper therapeutic equivalents
- rate of prescribing of drugs in certain defined therapeutic areas where overprescribing is known to occur (e.g. minor respiratory illness).

In summary, while crude prescribing rates and costs are certainly a poor indicator of quality in prescribing, and the notion of a capitation-based 'formula' for calculation of prescribing budgets according to need is controversial, there is theoretical justification for the development of generic prescribing rates and the prescription of certain 'marker' drugs as quality indicators in the field of prescribing. Further research in this area is currently being undertaken.

The topic-based perspective: measuring the overall quality of care in particular conditions

Management of specific acute episodes of organic illness, and the ongoing care of chronic conditions, both lend themselves to the standard principles of quality monitoring developed in the secondary care sector. Although it would not be valid to take such hospital-based quality-monitoring protocols 'off the peg' (since both the prevalence and the severity of illness and the ease of access to investigations differ between primary and secondary care), most clinicians would uphold the general principle of equal standards of care wherever care is delivered.

Although consensus statements suggesting quality standards are becoming ubiquitous in the medical literature, there are few conditions for which such standards can be defended as truly evidence-based. The current reality is often a combination of expert consensus, *a priori* reasoning, and research trial evidence. Professor Martin Roland and colleagues in Manchester are currently engaged in a large-scale initiative to develop consensus quality criteria for key chronic conditions using the Delphi method (Mays & Pope 1996).

The growing popularity of evidence-based medicine has brought a perception (and an expectation) that the management of particular conditions in primary care should be undertaken according to guidelines based on the best available research evidence. GPs frequently deal with ill-defined problems and what Murdoch (1997) called 'non-symptoms and non-disease', and the issue of appropriate guidelines which reflect the realities of primary care is a complex and controversial one. Although much speculation has been published on adherence to particular guidelines as a measure of quality of care by GPs, the success of such a venture in practice may be limited by political and cultural resistance from practitioners.

The professional perspective: education and development of GPs

Earlier chapters have highlighted the risk to GPs of professional isolation, disillusionment and burnout. One increasingly significant source of distress is the inability to keep abreast of developments in medical knowledge, especially the results and implications for practice of clinical research trials. This task is now impossible without protected time for study, a systematic approach to the published literature, access to electronic databases, and specific skills in critical appraisal. There is some evidence that doctors who have been trained in problem-based learning remain more up to date, effective and safe in their practice than those trained in traditional didactic methods (Sackett, Haynes, Guyatt, Tugwell 1994).

Research is currently under way evaluating the effectiveness of training in evidence-based practice in terms of patient-relevant outcomes. A programme of postgraduate education through personal learning plans and a lifelong, flexible strategy of personal development have been proposed for general practice, but there is currently no measurable aspect of practice or learning style which has been shown to be a reliable indicator of a high quality or evidence-based approach to practice. Thus, indicators of quality in professional education remain focused on the following:

- **Degrees and diplomas:** postgraduate examinations, RCGP fellowship by assessment, certification or accreditation in particular topics (e.g. minor surgery)

- **Attendance on courses:** postgraduate educational allowance approved courses for GPs, approved courses for practice nurses, training schemes for practice staff, practice-based multidisciplinary education programmes
- **Professional development:** attachments to academic departments of primary care, clinical assistantships in hospitals
- **Education through audit:** participation of practice-based audit and associated educational initiatives organised either through local medical (or multidisciplinary) audit advisory groups (MAAGs) or via academic links.

The manager's view: measuring the quality of teamwork in a multidisciplinary service organisation

Health authorities are increasingly concerned with the functioning of multidisciplinary teams in primary care, and failure to achieve clinical objectives may be ascribed to poor teamwork. Most studies of this area cannot be generally applied, or have examined single issues such as the effect of teamwork on the detection and management of hypertension.

The objective of primary care should not be teamwork *per se* but personalised care from a single practitioner coupled where appropriate with task-focused activity by ad hoc groups of staff with specific skills. The growing interest in measures of team functioning for primary care 'teams' should perhaps be modified by consideration of the wider literature on teamworking in general.

Conclusion: implications for the education–service partnership

There are no easy answers to the question 'How do we measure quality in general practice?'. Instruments developed in response to the objectives of one particular interest group may not serve the purposes of other groups. Perspectives on quality can and do conflict across different professions. The danger of the false objectivity engendered by one-dimensional numerical estimates of quality should be recognised and this approach resisted.

The education–service partnership in general practice is, at this stage, largely a theoretical construct which anticipates both collaboration across disciplines and the integration of different roles within particular individuals. We predict that strategy for implementing this initiative, and the negotiation of suitable markers of quality against which its success can be evaluated, will require the adoption of multiple paradigms. To this end, we would argue that the composition of key bodies such as MAAGs and the regional education boards, should explicitly reflect a wide range of different perspectives, including those of purchasers, secondary care, primary care, academia and service users.

Rather than attempting to produce a single, unitary measure of quality for evaluating 'the effect of the education–service partnership on primary care', these bodies should accept the reality of multiple paradigms and use the instruments referred to in this paper, and others where appropriate, as a toolkit with which to adopt a flexible, hypothesis-driven approach to specific questions. For example, the question 'what is the effect of the education–service partnership on referral rates to outpatient clinics?' will require a different set of tools from the question 'what is its effect on patients' perceptions of confidentiality?' or 'what is its effect on GP professional development?'.

References

Audit Commission (1994). *A prescription for improvement: towards more rational prescribing in general practice*. London: HMSO

Bosanquet N, Leese B (1995). Change in general practice and its effects on service provision in areas with different socioeconomic characteristics. *British Medical Journal* 311:546–50

British Thoracic Society (1997). The British guidelines on asthma management 1995 review and position statement. *Thorax* 52: Suppl 1:S1–S20

Elkin R, Robinson J (1997). Performance indicators as a source of motivation. In: Kennings S, Pringle M for the Working Group on Primary and Community Care Monitoring. *Effective purchasing of primary and community health care: promotion of quality in the provision of primary care*. Trent Institute for Health Services Research, Discussion Paper 97/01 (see Appendix D, pp38–55)

Evan M, Sweeney K (1998). *The human side of medicine*. Occasional Paper 76. London: RCGP

Greenhalgh T (1998). Calculating GP prescribing budgets; effective prescribing at practice level can and should be identified and rewarded. *BMJ* 316:750

Howie JGR, Porter AMD, Heaney DJ *et al*. (1991). Long to short consultation ratio: a proxy measure of quality of care for general practice. *British Journal of General Practice* 41:48–54

Howie JGR, Porter AMD, Heaney DJ *et al*. (1991). Attitudes to medical care, the organisation of work and stress among general practitioners. 42:181–5

Majeed A, Head S (1998). Capitation based prescribing budgets will not work. *BMJ* 316:748–53

Mays N, Pope C (1996). Qualitative methods in health research. BMJ publications. London: HMSO

Murdoch JC (1997). Mackenzie's puzzle – the cornerstone of teaching and research in general practice. *British Journal of General Practice* 47:656–8

Pereira Gray D (1992). *Planning primary care*. Occasional Paper 57. London: RCGP

Sackett DL, Haynes RB, Guyatt GH, Tugwell (1994). *Clinical epidemiology – basic science for clinical medicine*. London: Little Brown and Co.

Smith CH, Armstrong D (1989). Comparison of criteria derived by government and patients for evaluating general practitioner services. *BMJ* 299:494–6

Chapter 6

Developing strategy – views from the key players

This chapter reflects the personal views of people involved in education and service in general practice. There are similarities in the issues which they think are important, although the line they take often differs. Key issues identified include the following.

Why is there a need to change?

Kelly and Fuller highlight the professional requirements for involving patients.

Pietroni and Kilcoyne express the view that education and training changes lag behind practice changes which in turn lag behind policy changes.

Boyd suggests that policy changes lag behind long-term social, demographic and technological changes.

Several of the contributors highlight the growing emphasis on multidisciplinary or multiprofessional working in primary care. The manager and nurse contributors highlight clinical governance as another driving force for change.

The complex funding and organisational arrangements are described variously by the contributors as a 'shambles' (Boyd, as head of a medical school), a 'nightmare' and an 'opportunity' (Williams, the manager).

Why is change difficult?

Some of the difficulty certainly lies in the complexity of the existing arrangements. However, deeper reasons are given. Kelly and Fuller suggest that underlying the practical difficulty of involving patients in medical education in general practice is a fundamental issue of attitude: they are not regarded as partners but as subjects. Bolger, from a nursing perspective, suggests that GPs as doctors are taught to value their own skills and knowledge above others, and as proprietors of small businesses, focus on the business potential of education. Gilley, from the BMA's GP Committee, sees education as promoted too much from a punitive perspective rather than in a positive way.

All the contributors refer, at least implicitly, to a real or perceived conflict between education and service. Boyd suggests that it is a conflict between investing in current services and investing in future services. Gilley suggests it is a conflict about who pays for education. Williams also emphasises the issues around the priorities for use of scarce resources.

What is to be done?

The contributors generally agree that institutional barriers have to be removed and that practitioners (GPs and nurses in particular) need to be central to planning and delivering education. There is some consensus about the merits of practice or team-based education and training focused around clinical issues. Bolger, Pietroni and Kilcoyne are specific about things that need to done. Kelly and Fuller, Williams and Bolger give examples of good practice.

Success?

A number of contributors consider how the effectiveness of education will be measured. Williams talks about the NHS Executive performance indicators; Gilley discusses GP satisfaction; Boyd reflects on responding to changes over a potential career of 60 years. Kelly and Fuller look at changes in knowledge, skills and attitudes from a number of perspectives.

The Patient's Perspective
Diana Kelly and Jon Fuller

Why is change needed?

Patients have always been involved in medical education, but generally passively. They have been used as clinical material or training fodder to enable students to practise their skills of physical examination and history taking – this has been true in both a hospital and general practice setting.

Some people have been trained as simulated patients for the education or assessment of medical students (Barrows, 1971). Their role has however been tightly controlled by a clinical teacher. There is generally no opportunity for patients to apply their experience and expertise. Patients are generally treated as 'diseases', not people with lives before and beyond the medical setting. They are generally treated as 'teaching subjects' with medical staff and students in hospitals gathering round the bed and over the patient's recumbent body (Neuberger, 1998).

The General Medical Council (1993) has stressed the importance of medical students being able to understand patients within the context of their families and environment and also the importance of medical students being able to communicate effectively with both patients and carers. Developing the role of patients as educators is a means to achieve those ends.

The NHS Executive gave a high profile to collaboration with patients through the conference on 'Patient Partnership – What's in it for me?' in May 1997. Medical education should follow this lead.

What patients have to offer

Patients and carers have the potential to play much more than a passive role in medical education and the enhancement of their teaching role is long overdue. They have a special expertise and perspective about their health or ill health and the factors affecting it. By drawing on this, students not only improve their knowledge and understanding, but they can also enhance their communication skills and develop an attitude that respects the patient's perspective and the patient's rights.

Patients offer their considerable knowledge and the potential to facilitate students' learning. However, each patient may exercise this ability in a different way by offering different learning opportunities. If asked, patients have views on what they believe it is important for medical students to learn (for example, cultural and religious issues) and how they believe they can teach students about what it is actually like to live with illness or to care for somebody with a particular condition. Patients can also be involved in assessing the work of medical students and they should play a part in evaluating any training programme. Developing an educational partnership with patients involves consideration of issues such as support and training to enable full participation and accreditation as well as financial remuneration to recognise patients' unique contribution.

Why is change so difficult?

Teaching within general practice faces many challenges, which include the tension between service delivery and teaching and the difficulty of 'having the right patient with the right problem in the right place at the right time'. This illustrates the point that patients are expected to fit in with the students' timetable and agenda, with relatively little flexibility.

What is to be done?

To achieve the GMC's goals of seeking patients in context and communicating effectively, patients need to be involved not just as individuals but also through groups of patients and carers.

There is good practice already. In the USA there are a growing number of examples of a shift towards encouraging patients to use their personal experience and play a more active role in medical education. Weisser (1985) encouraged patients to adopt an active role in the conduct and direction of student seminars and students reported that this enabled them to consider the patient's problems in a broader context. Gruppen *et al.* (1996) trained people with arthritis to teach students to perform a whole body joint examination. They reported that this use of patients was highly effective in changing students' knowledge and attitudes. Vail *et al.* (1996) trained patients from an HIV group to teach interviewing, physical examination and counselling skills.

In the UK, medical education lags behind somewhat but, even so, some community-based programmes include family or patient attachments (for example, Fox, Joesbury & Hannay, 1991; Pill & Tapper-Jones, 1993). These provide an opportunity for students to visit patients in their homes. Here the student spends time with someone selected by a doctor who is usually the teacher of the programme. These attachments usually involve students using the patient and their family as a source of information, discussing their observations and exploring what they learn with the doctor rather than the patient.

Success

The examples above illustrate the kinds of measure of success in involving patients. They include changes in knowledge and attitudes, skills and confidence of medical students as measured by themselves, by patients and by other measurement tools.

PATIENTS AS PARTNERS – AN EXAMPLE OF GOOD PRACTICE

Between 1993 and 1996 the King's Fund supported an innovative experiential, community-based programme which was developed at St. Bartholomew's and the Royal London School of Medicine and Dentistry (Kelly, 1997). The Patients as Partners programme enabled over 100 patients to participate in a scheme whereby each spent up to a term with a medical student. Within the overall programme, opportunities were created by the 'patient partners' to address the students' self-determined learning needs. The students spent time with their patient partners in a variety of settings, both medical (e.g. general practice) and non-medical (e.g. at a tenants' association meeting to learn about the links between bad housing and health). The programme acknowledged the potential role of the patients as experts, facilitators, assessors and evaluators. Patient partners also encouraged students to meet with others involved in their care, such as home helps, district nurses, educational psychologists as well as relatives and friends. In addition, some suggested reading material for their students, which provided a contrast to the texts usually found on the students' reading lists.

The programme was successful from the point of view of the patients, students and tutors involved. Patients enjoyed taking part and felt that they had made a contribution to the training of future doctors. Patients also reported that they gained satisfaction from working collaboratively with students in their learning and from being active educators. The medical students who participated appear to have gained an understanding of their patient-partner's perspective, but the full impact of the programme may not be known for some time. An initial evaluation showed that the majority of medical students felt that their communication skills had improved and that they were more confident in talking with patients.

The potential for such a programme was realised by North Thames Postgraduate Medical and Dental Education who supported the development of the scheme at postgraduate level in the Department of Obstetrics and Gynaecology at Chelsea and Westminster Hospital. It is currently being extended to other specialisms within the hospital with the support of Chelsea and Westminster Healthcare Trust.

The Medical Perspective

Judy Gilley

We face a daunting challenge if we are to translate our brightest visions of an improved GP education system into functional and accessible structures for continuing professional development (CPD). We can only hope for success if the sort of joint working exemplified by the London Education and Service Partnership model is taken up across the board.

What do we mean by 'GP education'?

The term 'GP education' can be used as a shorthand for continuing professional development, in other words, for life-long learning which enables the individual GP to expand and fulfil their potential.

CPD is something of a catch-all encompassing a rich variety of modalities of GP continuing education, participation in audit, in research, and also the application of clinical effectiveness material.

The aims of GP education

We should be aiming for education for GPs which addresses the following headline themes, that is education which:

- provides a consistent source of professional satisfaction for GPs
- celebrates GPs' expertise
- demolishes barriers to participation
- dispels artificial boundaries
- generates enthusiasm for R&D
- encompasses the complexity of general practice
- attracts proper resources
- testifies to GPs' commitment to quality of services for patients.

Professional satisfaction

Professional satisfaction is fundamental because its nurturing is one route to the rekindling of the morale and confidence which general practice so urgently needs if it is to attract, and indeed to retain, the brightest and the best doctors. The 'from cradle to grave' educational model, spanning undergraduate days through to retirement, must be integral to the concept of being a GP, rather than an 'add on' activity. Of course, education must be self-directed. It must be adaptable to the increasingly complex ways in which GPs of the future will choose to work. It must cater for locums, retainees, returners, assistants and salaried GPs as well as principals. It should offer an attractive menu of exciting opportunities and should be made relevant to individual doctors, and to their practices. Every attempt should be made to provide education in ways which are effective.

Above all, the process must be enjoyable and provide, from time to time, the 'aha' of learning, the joy of making links in our understanding which really illuminate. It must be spiced with the excitement of discovery.

Celebrating GPs' expertise

Too often education has been perceived as something to be 'done' to GPs to make them better. The GP newspapers and even sometimes the 'serious' journals, as well as the non-generalists, special interest groups and some health authorities, all delight in telling GPs what they should be doing, what they are missing and where they should be directing their energies. However, rather than focusing on these negative and undermining messages, the emphasis should be on recognising and building on the cumulative expertise of the clinical generalist and on celebrating and analysing the supremely difficult daily juggling act which is general practice.

GPs live dangerously because they frequently tolerate uncertainty. In protecting patients from unnecessary investigations and in fulfilling their gatekeeper function GPs inevitably take risks. So while we should be receptive to evidence-based suggestions, our education must be self-directed. Most GPs know their own deficiencies as, sadly, one real expertise acquired during traditional medical education is the ability to disguise and protect one's weaknesses. What GPs of today need is the confidence to repeatedly challenge themselves.

Education is too often seen as a commodity, part of the enterprise culture with too much emphasis on problem-solving and too much of a procedural ring. We need to build on the understandings and skills gained in GP vocational training and in GPs' participation in teaching students, particularly understanding about how adults learn. Like all students, GPs needs to ask themselves: 'What sort of learning works best for me?'; 'What constitutes a good learning experience for me?'; 'Who, or what, facilitated my learning?' We need to build on the best of the LIZEI schemes (see Chapter 3).

The barriers to participation

We must slay the dragon of anxiety about 'being found wanting'. Although all GPs need excellent continuing professional development, only a very small percentage are seriously wanting and exhibit deficient performance needing remedial help. The profession shares the Government's concern to ensure patient safety and supports the General Medical Council's 'poor performance procedures' as well as the recently enhanced responsibilities of health authorities for the prevention of under-performance. However, we must not let these important responsibilities generate counterproductive anxiety about participation in education for the average GP. GP education must not be a source of professional pain, otherwise it is doomed. It must also continue to be professionally led.

Service and education

Barriers between service commitments and education must go. Education must fit into the working week comfortably as an integral part of a GP's working life, carried out in protected time.

> LIZEI 'free up Thursday' schemes where the local GP co-operative was used to cover surgeries so that doctors were able to pursue their own professional development one half-day a week could form a model.

Institutional barriers

Barriers also need to be demolished to allow the functional integration of undergraduate and postgraduate educational structures. Barriers between teaching and learning as well as between learners and teachers also need to crumble because the best teachers are also actively learning. Barriers and hostility between academics and non-academics work to the detriment of general practice. LIZEI education boards with membership from local medical committees, undergraduate and postgraduate education interests and health authorities have demonstrated the strength of learning to work together.

Promoting multidisciplinary education

Barriers to multidisciplinary education, especially at practice level, also need to be eroded. This facet of the educational spectrum needs to be developed to improve teamworking and joint management of patient care.

Priorities for education

Putting research into practice

We need to provide future GPs with better evidence on the many topics which form part of the current R&D programme, for example, on how best to investigate chest pain presenting in general practice, on the outcomes of influenza and pneumococcal immunisation and on screening for postnatal depression.

Catering for the complexity of general practice

Education needs to encompass knowledge base, skills, professional attitudes, organisation of services, use of clinical effectiveness and participation in the complex ethical issues of practice. General practice is not only a science, but also a 'humanist activity concerned with human relationships'. Yet education is all too often dominated by a tightly knotted knowledge system which excludes the social sciences and the humanities. We need to foster a wider vision.

Attracting proper resources

Education needs to be resourced both in the human terms of skilled educationalists and the professional 'shapers' and in the sense of the financial underpinning of its structures, including support for protected time for GP participation.

How much education?

How much time is it appropriate for GPs to spend on education? The current postgraduate educational accreditation (PGEA) system supports half an hour a week. The last workload survey indicated that GPs spend approximately two hours a week in all educational activities, including travelling to participate. The gold standard should be in the order of half a day a week.

Protect pay while promoting professionalism

The funding sources for GP education are currently complex as are all parts of the GP pay system. PGEA is part of 'intended average gross remuneration' and is regarded by GPs as part of their pay. There have been many criticisms of the current PGEA system and many GPs and others wish to see it replaced by a professionally led form of CPD. PGEA funds would have to be returned to the pool and there would need to be full funding for a new system. There is broad support for the conclusion of the Government's consultation exercise on professional development that 'in the NHS education and training is an investment not a cost'.

The General Practice Committee wishes to see its reaccreditation policy forwarded through pilots with a view to successful schemes being taken up nationally in due course. There would need to be a PGEA equivalent paid to GPs who volunteered to participate in reaccreditation pilots. Eventually, the current PGEA system would wither on the vine.

Providing high-quality patient services

All GPs want to achieve the best for their patients. Education which enhances knowledge about medicine and use of services, and understanding of the individual patient leads to improved decision-making by both the doctor and patient and ultimately to health gain for the patient. Health gain is therefore the meeting ground of the education and service responsibilities of GPs.

The Academic Perspective

Robert Boyd

A distinguished trust chairman, Lord Glenarthur, remarked in a House of Lords debate that we cannot have the 'academic tail' wagging the 'service dog'. However, this is based on a misreading of the nature of the interface between the academic and service for reasons given below.

What is education for?

The academic is the 'futures' element of service care provision. Care depends on the service but moving through a generation of young people there will not be a service, or no service of quality, unless that academic element is injected over the years. The timescale is long. The agenda is 30 or 60 years. Young people deciding what A levels to do today, and whether to go into medicine or nursing, are going to be in full flight of practice in the middle of the next century. It is inevitable that the retirement age will move up, and today's young people may well not be giving up their professional career until about the year 2062.

Education for change

The academic perspective should focus on educating the young, inspiring the middle-aged, reflecting on our practice and using that reflection to innovate and change and reflect more deeply (which we call research). This gives us the flexibility to cope with change.

New bioscience and information technology brings new possibilities: being able to study a patient's genes and predicting whether they are likely to develop Alzheimer's disease, for example.

The rise in the dependent population must be seen in the context of low taxation – the individual's choice in how to spend their money is very much on the agenda at the moment. We have a very unstable equilibrium and anything could happen – we may be struck by a meteor, we might suffer social discohesion, or we may go to war. It is important not to make too many assumptions.

Personnel issues

Another question mark hangs over the staffing context. The rise of multiprofessionalism is increasing the expectation of our young people over career satisfaction. We have seen major morale problems in primary care in the last five to ten years. We are still very unused to people making career changes in medicine but in future people will move in and out of medicine and in and out of specialties. People also want a domestic life and partnerships tend not to survive when one partner is a workaholic.

A complex picture

We have a complicated brew of undergraduate education, postgraduate and continuing professional development and R&D. The whole system works only fairly badly at the teaching hospital campus with all its different academic agendas.

For example, St George's Hospital is a campus with a medical school on one corner with a big teaching hospital adjacent to it. About £210m is spent there per year. About two-thirds is current patient services and about one-third is 'futures', i.e. education, research and development. The total futures spend is considerably bigger than the medical school spend. It includes Higher Education Funding Council fees, NHS spend (staff paid by investment the NHS has made directly for chairs etc. and the R&D stream), commercial and charitable contracts, plus European Union monies.

In addition, on the NHS-side there is the service increment for teaching (SIFT), the postgraduate medical and dental education levy (MADEL), non-medical education and training (NMET) and the R&D budget. That is the brew and the reason it works at all is because there are formal structures from government downwards. There is the standing group on undergraduate medical and dental education. There are also ten key principles, signed up to by the Secretary of State for Health, concerning how the two halves should work together. Trust representatives sit on the medical school council, people from the schools sit on various trust councils, and there are relations with the health authority. It all amounts to 'biographical glue' – individual people engaged in teaching, in research, in clinical care.

The primary care dimension

In comparison with the above, primary care is an absolute shambles. You have medical schools, independent general practice with its various subsets, community trusts, as well as the other primary care elements – opticians, dentists and social workers. And if it is hard enough to get a futures perspective within a teaching hospital campus, then imagine how difficult it is to achieve a shared vision with all those disparate players, despite the stunning areas of achievement in some areas, notably postgraduate education and training in general practice. When you have 272 individual practices on different sites, plus all the other professions involved, it makes it very difficult to achieve the futures vision.

Barriers to change

The future is ours and perhaps the education consortia will help us to deliver it. The constraints include the following:

- limited number of GPs with the time to engage in these futures activities
- poor levels of facilities funding
- the weakness of the interface with the wider medical school
- myths and ignorance in the teaching hospitals/disease palaces. For instance, the idea that if you can get the students out into primary care, that is where they are going to see multidisciplinary working! Sometimes it works brilliantly but we must not lose sight of the reality of many primary care teams
- the fragmented funding streams, the different management agendas, the regulatory and legal boundaries moving money from one stream to another
- the problems for the individual practitioner. We are pushed for money, pushed for time and pulled in different directions
- the research assessment exercise
- the misconception that general practice means 'touchy feely' teamwork rather than intellectually demanding decision-making.

The strength of what we can do in primary care is obvious. The future belongs to GPs. They are having a big impact on undergraduate medical teaching.

In conclusion

The strength of what we can do in primary care is obvious. The future belongs to GPs. Thay are having a big impact on undergraduae medical teaching but it is clear that three-year timescales are inadequate. As for Lord Glenarthur's dog, the tail and the body are one and we need to work to make that a harmonious reality.

The Manager's Perspective

Susan Williams

Of the total Tomlinson LIZ funding of some £460m, around £10m was spent on education. Before the inception of LIZ, in the late 1980s/early 1990s, general medical services received fewer resources. Health Authorities spent between £30,000 and £40,000 per year on training, principally for practice nurses, practice receptionists and practice managers. GPs could attend lectures at a local postgraduate centre, if they had one. Lecturers were hospital consultants in white coats, lunch was provided by a drug company and PGEA approval was sought.

The impact of Tomlinson

The legacy of Tomlinson was considerable new money for education in a district like Barking & Havering. In 1993/94 the training budget was £35,000. With LIZ a sum of £796,000 became available over three years. It was difficult to spend such increased sums.

In Barking and Dagenham, where we had the funding, we have tried to ensure engagement of the average GP. We established an education board, building on a postgraduate education group which had been reviewing the way postgraduate education was traditionally delivered. We took the opportunity of directing the funding to this ready-made group of interested individuals. The Local Medical Committee was included in these discussions. We were keen to ensure there was a gender balance and also a geographical balance. We have invested in developing an academic unit. We have been working with the university medical school to set up lecturer posts there in the hope that they will form the basis of R&D capacity. As managers, we have tried to assist, guide and support the education board and its members. Our role is to sort out the funding. We have encouraged people to come forward with their own ideas.

Results

The board built up a programme based on needs identified by the group in Barking and Dagenham. A large range of opportunities have come from this funding. Of the 76 eligible GPs all but three have been engaged in some kind of activity. Mentoring has been particularly successful. In the early days people were very nervous about it. The experience of mentoring was stressful in itself. Building in mutual support is important for handling the role. Discussion groups are flourishing in centres around Barking and Dagenham. This has led to less hostility towards the health authority and to managers in general.

How do managers begin to judge these kinds of initiative?

Performance indicators – These are limited and it is problematic linking changes to investment
Morale and well-being of doctors – It is important to overcome isolation and low self-esteem

The consortia present new roles for all of us. Previously, managers had a choice: if you were interested in education then you became involved; otherwise, you did not. There is now a new expectation of managers, many of whom have not got the measure of this task yet. The huge range of potential funding sources is confusing. There is a great deal of work for HAs, working with GPs, to understand these funding sources and to ensure a budget for primary care education.

The future

Primary care groups are going to be managing large budgets with large responsibilities. We have therefore forged links with postgraduate educationalists for a development programme for PCG members. We are trying to maintain a sizeable programme in the face of a £2m deficit with the trusts. Support for clinical governance is crucial. The prospect of being personally accountable for the clinical quality of the consultants or GPs means that, if managers have not taken an interest in education before, they certainly will now. Closer contact should ensure a closer correspondence between funding and results.

To promote team-based development we have extended our education board to include practice nursing and practice management.

Conclusion

Involvement in education and training is no longer a choice for managers. Chief executives are expected to ensure that HAs have the capability to handle this agenda. The manager's role is to:

- understand how one gains access to this money
- help and support the education board
- make linkages across the system – health authorities have a responsibility to bring secondary care and primary care together
- work with boroughs to create an integrated learning environment
- spot opportunities for funding (e.g. European or joint finance) and make sure the educationalists have access to these sources of funding
- create a climate of support. This is about giving GPs a sense of confidence, building a sense of trust in the HA. Practitioners must feel able to come forward with ideas and proposals to meet their educational needs.

The Nurse's Perspective

Tom Bolger

Recognising the need and opportunity for change

It is encouraging that there now seems to be a widespread acceptance that general practice needs to take education seriously. In the past many doctors have been happy with a PGEA system which allows them to go along to the postgraduate medical centre, enjoy a lunch provided by a drug company and hear a consultant give a lecture. They met their PGEA requirements and it cost them nothing except their time. Indeed many remain happy with this system.

However, the advent of new funding systems like MADEL and NMET have broadened people's thinking and there appears to be a general recognition that the new approach offers new opportunities which should make education more widely available. Sadly, the 'small business' mentality of some doctors has led them to focus on the potential for income generation through providing education, for example, by seeking to charge for student placements in practices. LIZEI money prompted them to start thinking about what it was costing them to educate themselves and what they could charge for educating others.

MADEL, NMET and other sources of income should act as an external motivating force to encourage people to access education. It does not matter whether GPs see education as a useful way of keeping the business going through charging for providing education, or whether they view it as a necessary investment in order to keep the practice going. Either way, the commitment to education is there.

Tensions between doctors and nurses

Practice nurses are keen to broaden their skills but in some areas they are not being allowed to do this. GPs seem reluctant to help nurses gain more qualifications unless it directly benefits the practice, but this is leading to frustration for some nurses and is affecting morale.

Practice nurses do not want to feel they have to go cap in hand to their GP when they want education and there needs to be a recognition among all doctors that times are changing. Nurses are now employing doctors in personal medical services pilot schemes, such as those in Derby and Salford. Of course, nurses have commissioned GP services for years in nursing homes and also in nurse-led units in hospitals. In that respect any perceived challenge to medical dominance is not new. But these developments should not be viewed as a threat because there are so many common elements to the needs of the whole team when it comes to education.

Meanwhile, it seems that the advent of PCGs is causing disquiet among GPs, some of whom also regard this new development as a threat. They see their own individual clinical practice being challenged with people like nurses becoming involved in decision-making on how practices are run. Changes are happening quickly, and it will be interesting to see how the new system beds down, but paternalism is out and power-sharing is in.

If care is to be patient-centred, community-centred, citizen-centred, or whatever buzz words you choose, then autocratic behaviour on the part of doctors will not do. It is important to engender a team approach, recognising that what each member has to offer is important and relevant. Each person's contribution must be respected.

Life-long learning

Another significant external drive in education is the growing recognition of the importance of life-long learning, not just in health care but across industry and in society in general. If, as predicted, people are going to have three or four different careers in a lifetime, then they will need to learn and develop all the time in order to move from one role to another.

Mandatory continuing education

Another external force that has come into play is the realisation that for doctors, mandatory continuing education is on the cards. It is already a reality for nurses and practices now have to release nurses for continuing education in order to enable them to stay on the register. If nurses are needed in the primary health care team, as of course they are, then the team must look at ways of ensuring they are able to keep themselves up to date.

Clinical governance

The introduction of clinical governance will alter how every clinician and manager in the NHS is held accountable for their actions. This will inevitably lead to health authorities and the PCGs taking more of an interest in what is going on behind GPs' doors than has been the case in the past.

It will also make GPs and nurses far more motivated to get it right when it comes to education, keeping up to date and focusing on what is effective. Education within a general practice should, as a bottom line, improve the health of the people for whom the service is provided. And while it might be difficult to make a direct link between good professional education and health gain among the public, there must be enough circumstantial evidence which says there is such a link. Education is no longer an option. It is now part of the business.

What sort of education do we need?

Education has to have certain inherent values and one key tenet is respect for one another. There is a need to respect the differences as well as the similarities between members of the team. If you start from this premise, you can then look at the best ways of providing education and training and the best ways of structuring the learning programme itself.

Acknowledging differences means you need not expect education to be delivered to everybody in the same room at the same time. For instance, if you were addressing the need for updating in pharmacology, you might say, 'This is what the doctors need to know and this is what the nurses need'. It follows that if there is mutual respect, then if a doctor was looking at diabetes or epilepsy, for example, she or he might say, 'I wonder if the nurse knows more about this than I do?'

Each member of the primary care team is engaged in some degree of diagnostic work. They are the first point of contact for the public, therefore in any consideration of the content of educational programmes, sharpening people's diagnostic skills must feature quite highly. Similarly, many different members of the team will be involved in health promotion.

The content of educational programmes could be focused on diseases, services or client groups. For instance, in a practice that runs clinics for asthma, family planning, leg ulcers, diabetes, well-woman and well-man sessions, everybody involved in the practice would have to be updated on all of this but individuals may need more advanced development if they take a lead role in any particular field.

How do you deliver education?

One of the central problems in education comes from those who organise it. They have tended to expect people to come to them, or go to a centre, to access learning, when what people want is something more flexible.

They want to determine their own pace of learning and they want choice. Above all, they want much of their education to happen in the workplace.

When considering all this, it is important to think about the delivery system: who can do the teaching and who can say that it is being done properly. There are three points to bear in mind:

- the relevant people within the team need to have expertise and be responsible for structuring the learning programmes
- it is important to look at the technology available, including the Internet, CD-ROM, video, distance-learning packages, etc.
- external bodies should be involved who can provide validated materials and who will audit the system.

For nurses, bodies such as the Royal College of Nursing and the English National Board approve such schemes. The medical royal colleges are also beginning to become more involved in this area.

Having access to accredited materials offers people more choice, and distance learning enables people to create the space in their professional life to reflect on what is going on. This reflection can take place either individually or in teams. Practice meetings are one forum. However, currently, they do not always include all members of the team.

The Primary Health Care Team's Perspective

Patrick Pietroni and Anne Kilcoyne

Changing service needs

The population now lives longer. NHS resources are shifting away from the treatment of acute illnesses to the treatment of chronic illnesses and their long-term management. The locus of care of people with long-term illness is shifting from the hospital setting into the community. This has called for a re-assessment of the purpose, working methods, structure and staffing of general practice.

The volume of policy statements encouraging interprofessional working arrangements has been increasing in recent years, with the NHS and Community Care Act 1990, the White Papers, *Delivering the Future* (1996), *A Service with Ambitions* (1996), *Choice and Opportunity* (1996), and the Primary Health Care Act 1997. At breath-taking speed, the previous Conservative government decreed that much of what used to be the province of the single-handed GP practice, the psychiatric and geriatric hospital, as well as the post-operative nursing service of the general hospital, was to become the territory of the primary health care team working in a multiservice health centre alongside community care, social services, pharmaceutical and dental services.

The new NHS White Paper (1997) builds on this policy trend. In fact, the concepts of collaboration, co-operation and integrated working across boundaries, sectors and agencies are extended through PCGs. These represent the health needs of between 47,000 and 270,000 patients and are led by GPs. They will be responsible for commissioning health services from hospitals (and as primary care trusts for providing community services). They will work in partnership with health authorities to develop and commission the resources for Health Improvement Plans. The call for collaboration and co-operation is indeed imperative.

Practice, of course, always lags behind policy. The nature and structure of the primary health care team varies enormously from practice to practice. There are still many single-handed GPs, particularly in inner city areas. These GPs are now obliged to join PCGs and to work collaboratively. The primary health care team can comprise any number of doctors in both partnership and non-partnership contractual arrangements. There may be several nursing professionals attached to the practice – the practice nurse, the nurse practitioner, the health visitor, the midwife and/or the community nurse. There is often a practice manager. Other ancillary professionals such as physiotherapists, osteopaths, counsellors, etc. may be brought into the team according to the service needs and aspirations of the practice. The community pharmacist and dentist are also part of the primary care network and in some health centres are already integrated into the organisation.

Interprofessional training needs

Just as practice lags behind policy, so education and training lags behind practice. Health service providers, particularly in the primary care sector, are having to manage an enormous amount of change in a complex organisational field in a very short time. These processes of change have produced in many professionals a sense of confusion, overload, frustration, anxiety and, for some, burn-out. It is not enough to throw professionals together and let them make the most of it. The organisational and collaborative strategies which these service changes call for need support, training and education.

Working within a multiprofessional team dealing with life and death issues calls for high levels of competence and mutual respect. Differential pay and hierarchical relationships do not easily translate into flexible, task-oriented teamworking. All too often the primary health care team is marked by tribal behaviours, each profession prioritising its own vested interests, each employing different languages, value systems, philosophies and approaches to the care of patients.

Nevertheless, the thrust towards collaboration has thrown up some innovative service delivery and education. Where there has been such leadership, the 'seamless service delivery' called for in the 1996 White Paper, *A Service with Ambitions*, has been achieved. Where a spirit of collaboration has informed the processes of change, job satisfaction and fellowship in work have increased. Normally, burdensome workloads plagued by dysfunctional communication patterns and sticky working structures can be improved. Gaps in service delivery across agency interfaces and costly cross-disciplinary repetitions in procedures can be avoided. Collaborative work should involve carers' representatives and the different perspectives of users themselves.

Evaluation of different models of interprofessional working in different settings has been patchy and further research, development and audit are called for. The mistaken perceptions and professional stereotypes that impede interprofessional work are best addressed through shared learning around real practice problems. This generates shared understanding, language and values that facilitate collaboration. Training opportunities that include a range of workers from different agencies and different organisational levels need to take account of differing timetables. Early good examples of interagency collaboration help to demonstrate the 'art of the possible'. A broad range of teaching methods are required with particular emphasis on experiential learning to best illustrate the complexity of interprofessional working.

Individual professionals need skills in communication, both written and oral, formal and informal. A range of leadership skills are required to complete multi-agency teams and networks. Finally, they need stress management skills!

References

Barrows HS (1971). *Simulated patients*. Springfield (IL): Charles C. Thomas

Fox NJ, Joesbury H, Hannay DR (1991). Family attachments and medical sociology; a valuable partnership for students learning. *Medical Education* 25:155–9

General Medical Council (1993). *Tomorrow's doctors: recommendations on undergraduate medical education*. London: General Medical Council

Gruppen LD, Branch VK, Laing TJ (1996). The use of trained patient educators with rheumatoid arthritis to teach medical students. *Arthritis Care and Research* 9(4):302–8

Kelly D (1997). Patients as partners in medical education. In: Whitehouse C, Roland M, Campion P (eds). *Teaching Medicine in the Community*. Oxford: Oxford University Press

Neuberger J (1998). The patient's perspective: a challenge for medical education. In: Jolly B, Rees L. *Medical education in the millennium*. Oxford: Oxford University Press

Pill RM, Tapper-Jones LM (1993). An unwelcome visitor? The opinions of mothers involved in a community-based undergraduate teaching project. *Medical Education* 27:238–44

Vail R, Mahon-Salazar C, Morrison A, Kalet A. (1996). Patients as teachers: an integrated approach to teaching medical students about the ambulatory care of HIV infected patients. *Patient Education and Counselling* 27:95–101

Weisser RJ, Medio FJ (1985). The patient as teacher. *Journal of Medical Education* 60:63–5

Chapter 7

Education–service partnership: the route to a better future

Paul Wallace and Iona Heath

The LIZEI programme provided general practice in inner London with a unique three-year opportunity. For the first time, it was possible for GPs to give serious consideration to planning and undertaking further professional development, in the knowledge that they could be released from some clinical duties because resources were available to fund locum cover. Despite innumerable administrative and other problems, the programme acted as a powerful stimulus to general practice within the LIZ area (incidentally, causing a good deal of resentment amongst those excluded for geographical reasons), with more than 75 per cent of eligible GPs taking up one or more LIZEI-funded educational opportunity.

The programme was characterised by a rich diversity of activity and the level of involvement in LIZEI varied enormously between practices. Some GPs undertook only one or more short postgraduate training programmes, while others made major personal and professional commitments in studying for a master's degree, undertaking undergraduate teaching to medical students or transferring for a year or more to a university department as an academic fellow or a London Academic Training Scheme (LATS) trainee (Jones, Freeman 1998).

The programme offered a unique opportunity to explore ways in which the education–service partnership could be developed in general practice. It bolstered work already being undertaken in this direction in university departments of general practice and in the postgraduate organisations, and led to closer working relationships between these two educational sectors. Most importantly, it made it possible for GPs as individuals to give serious consideration to their personal educational needs, and to work within partnerships on important issues of practice development.

The following personal view of the potential of the education–service partnership is written from the perspective of a busy inner London general practice where one of us (IH) works. While this experience was unique, it was nonetheless typical of many similar practices in London, and we use it here to illustrate the ways in which involvement in the LIZEI programme had an impact on the education–service partnership in general practice.

Personal experience of the LIZEI experiment

The successes

LIZEI was wonderful: for the first time, hard-pressed GPs working in deprived and neglected areas had been given the time, space and resources to think creatively about their educational needs. All of the partners have benefited individually and, between us, we have learned:

- more about the use of computers in the practice
- the skills to take on more undergraduate training
- more about the dynamics of the consultation through membership of a Balint Group
- more about HIV and AIDS through attachment to a department of genito-urinary medicine.

The latter was such a success that one partner has since been taken on as a valued hospital practitioner within the department for one session a week, somewhat to the dismay of the remaining partners, although with great benefit to the practice's large number of HIV-positive patients. The practice also had the enormous good fortune to be the host for the clinical sessions of a LATS trainee who came for a year, for two clinical sessions a week, and used the practice patients as the basis for her research. The practice has always had a lot of enthusiasm for original research but had never actually achieved any. The experience of supporting the academic trainee through to a completed and published qualitative research project (Hoult 1998) gave extremely useful insights into the processes of research and made it all seem much more possible. The increased involvement of the practice in academic work in conjunction with the university department of primary care and population sciences resulted in it becoming one of the newly designated university-linked practices (ULP).

A doomed attempt at practice-based education

The above were the successes. Less satisfactory were the attempts of two partners to use LIZEI resources to develop a programme of genuinely practice-based education – a true education–service partnership. The local LIZEI overseers did their best to support the initiative, and provided locum cover for the doctors involved and an initial facilitated session to identify the learning needs which the primary health care team wished to prioritise. However, there was no support available to any other members of the team, and they were variously able to carve out the time from their usual work commitments.

Three half-day sessions were held, but with gradually falling attendance as the lack of proper infrastructure began to tell. Nonetheless, each session was judged a success by those able to attend, which included practice nurses, district nurses, health visitors, undergraduate medical students, GP registrars and GPs. The first was on epilepsy and focused on the failings of the practice's services to patients with epilepsy, perhaps particularly in terms of emotional support, and how these could be improved. The second was a wonderfully interactive session on wound management devised by the district nurses. They brought a large number of dressings and wound management products to the session. Many of the other members of the team knew of these only by name, and it was very useful to be able to handle the products while discussing their different properties.

The final session was led by the partner who had developed her expertise on HIV and AIDS, and participants each recounted the impact of their first encounter with patients ravaged by the HIV virus, all of whom had later died. The participants learned about the rapidly improving prognosis, and shared both optimism and fears for the future.

As an educational process it felt right, yet in the current circumstances it seemed doomed. The attempt was to ground education in the real challenges of the partners' daily working lives, bridging the gaps between areas of expertise to the benefit of individual patients known to all.

The practice as a learning organisation

Every practice is a learning organisation (see Chapter 4). Everyone whose working life brings them into contact with patients learns something new about life, health, illness and disease every day; we all of us learn most from our patients. Yet in present circumstances, this learning occurs by default and against the odds. The world is not divided between the good people who reflect on their practice, and the bad people who do not. Everybody reflects on what they do, but often in a very disorganised and unfocused way. When things are bad, we may learn more about survival skills than about how to do better for our patients. We work under pressure – for GPs this means a different patient at least every ten minutes. There is little time for refreshment, let alone reflection. Interprofessional issues are usually dealt with during a few precious minutes over coffee, and the wonder is that this works so well so often. Sharing coffee must be the greatest single promoter of teamworking. Yet space and time for proper reflection renews interest and enthusiasm, breeds new ideas and fosters both recruitment and retention.

Reflection is also infectious. What a shame that the present systems of education take people away from their patients and their colleagues for educational sessions which are still, despite the rhetoric, mostly confined to a single professional group. The gulf between service and education is built into the educational structure.

A better future

There are clear lessons from all of this about the importance of developing the education–service partnership to secure a better future, though the solutions as to how to build a programme to secure that better future are more complex. Increased involvement in postgraduate education and professional development must be one of the key goals of such a programme, accompanied by better opportunities to undertake undergraduate teaching of medical students. Such opportunities should ideally be extended to include involvement in primary care research.

The experience of the LIZEI programme has provided examples of the many different ways in which practices can undertake activities of this kind, and these can serve as a guide to the building of future programmes (see Chapter 3). Central to all of this is the need to enable GPs as individuals to give serious consideration to their personal educational needs, and to work within partnerships on important issues of practice development. For this to be possible, the concept of the education–service partnership as a key to primary care development must first be established. There needs to be recognition by all parties that the workload of a practice (not just the GPs) can be legitimately regarded as including not only clinical service commitments, but also involvement in professional development and academic work. If this is to prove possible, then equivalent financial incentives (accompanied by appropriate quality control mechanisms) will need to be established for the education component of the partnership. The 'Red Book' terms of service need to allow sufficient flexibility to enable the partnership to develop.

What does all of this mean at the level of the practice?

Protected time

Within the practice, one can argue for a complete transformation of postgraduate education, with regular educational sessions that are properly resourced taking place in each practice. A full half-day every two months would seem to be a good starting position. To achieve this, each primary health care team will need protected time for all its members (see Chapter 6). Protected time was one of the key elements that the LIZEI programme was able to provide, and possibly the single most important factor contributing to the success of the programme. Protected time can be achieved only by bringing into the practice additional workforce to undertake the clinical service provision which would normally be undertaken by the primary health care team members engaging in educational activity. During the LIZEI programme, this was achieved largely through employing locums, funded through the programme, to provide emergency medical cover. However, locums often proved difficult to find, and had the disadvantage of lack of familiarity with the practice and its patients. An alternative adopted by some practices was to use resources from LIZEI and academic departments to take on a clinical assistant, and in some cases additional administrative support. This had the advantage of continuity and integration of the new members of staff into an expanded primary health care team.

Information services

Each team will need the services of a clinical librarian and an educational facilitator, both of whom would attend every education session. The experience of LIZEI demonstrates that practice teams have little difficulty in identifying their learning needs; the problems come in deciding the order of priority for the range of needs that will always be identified. Significant event auditing could provide an accessible starting point. Expert facilitation is probably essential to ensure a proper balance between the educational needs of different members of the team, and to enable a sustained focus on meeting these. Both the facilitator and the librarian would be able to help the participants more effectively to wrestle with the two conundrums of evidence-based primary health care: the application of specialist research findings to generalist settings, and the application of population-based research findings to the care of individuals.

The aim is for each primary health care team to become an educationally facilitated learning set, and for all sessions to be accredited for continuing professional development by all the professional groups involved.

Involvement with academic departments

Building on this base, the resources of academic departments could be brought in to extend learning, for some or all of the members of the team, and enable the deeper reflection which becomes research. Opportunities should be extended for involvement in undergraduate teaching through programmes such as CeMENT, enabling GPs to update their knowledge and clinical skills through 'teaching the teacher' programmes and ongoing contact with medical students and hospital-based clinicians. Techniques of academic detailing could be appropriate to problem areas identified by the deliberations of the learning sets.

What must be done?

The maintenance and development of the bridges built during the LIZEI programme between primary health care teams, health services management at different levels, and academics in the undergraduate and postgraduate sector will be key for the growth of the education–service partnership. The natural vehicle for this will be PCGs which, while developing their involvement in issues relating to service development, will need to ensure the provision of support for educational activity.

PCGs must take on the issue of provision of protected time for primary health care teams to develop the education–service partnership. Although the LIZEI programme is no longer active, there is an increasing availability of NHS funds to support education and research in primary care, including SIFT, MADEL, NMETS and Culyer funds for research (see Chapter 2). PCGs can ensure that mechanisms are established to enable primary health care teams to have proper access to such funds, and to enable them to make adequate staffing provision to provide protected time that does not erode services to patients. This might include the development by PCGs of a pool of locums as well as mechanisms to enable practices to take on an additional clinical assistant or possibly a part-time partner. Clinical governance leads will need to ensure that nurses' educational interests are equally strongly represented (see Chapter 6).

GP tutors may play an important role within the PCG structure as part of the clinical governance sub-committee alongside the nurse tutor. Practice and professional assessment could be similar to the practice visits and peer review already carried out for assessment and re-approval of training practices. At a practice level, they would liaise with a practice education co-ordinator over the linkage between practice development training ('bottom-up agenda'), the PCG service development plan, the health improvement plan and national guidelines ('top-down agenda').

PCGs must have dedicated funding to provide sufficient skilled educational facilitators and clinical librarians, backed by access to academic libraries, to service regular practice meetings in each of their member practices. The team of educational facilitators and librarians must have clear links to academic departments so that these are able to respond to the identified educational needs.

University departments and postgraduate establishments, including the Royal College of General Practitioners, need to work closely with PCGs to ensure that involvement of primary health care teams in undergraduate education, postgraduate learning and research can develop synergistically. There will be many ways in which such synergy can be achieved, depending on the nature and the size of the practices. One such model is the University Linked Practice (ULP) which developed during the LIZEI programme, primarily to enable the development of substantial increases in community-based teaching of medical students and primary care research. For these practices, commitment to the education–service partnership constitutes a major part of the practice's work and their development was undertaken in close collaboration with universities and medical schools. This involvement in the university education and research enterprise is becoming increasingly important as expectations of primary care increase centrally within the NHS and medical academia. The LIZEI enabled a degree of collaboration on the development of ULPs which was unrivalled elsewhere in the UK. It enabled the development of premises and equipment (including information technology) and the provision of proper staffing, high-quality training opportunities, clear quality control mechanisms and the production of university contracts. The new primary care R&D networks provide another opportunity for cross-linking. While these developments are likely to be relevant for only a limited number of practices, they represent crucial steps in building the education–service partnership.

Those responsible for the accreditation of continuing professional development in each of the professional groups must ensure co-operative mechanisms of accrediting the activities of practice-based learning sets. They could also work closely with academics running 'teaching the teacher' programmes for general practice and undertaking quality control for undergraduate community-based medical education.

In this way we could achieve a genuine education–service partnership, with reflection and learning arising directly from the reality of the problems presented by patients, and the challenges which these pose to those charged with the delivery of health care services. Such education has the potential to reflect the breadth of primary health care and would be grounded on measures of quality which are perceived as valid by those, both patients and professionals, who find themselves at the sharp end. Such education would actively support service delivery, rather than undermine it, and that, above all, must be our shared ambition.

References

Hoult L (1998). Why do patients call out-of-hours following a recent consultation with their GP? A qualitative study in one general practice. *Fam Pract* 15; Supplement 1:S30–S35

Jones R, Freeman G (eds) (1998). The London Academic Training Scheme (LATS). *Fam Pract* 15; Supplement 1

Wallace P, Drage S, Jackson N (1998). Linking education and service in general practice. *BMJ* 316:323.

Primary care – a partnership between education and the service in London North Thames

A joint statement from the representatives of the London Medical Schools (RFH/UCL), the Deans of Postgraduate General Practice and the LIZ Task Force

Three themes have dominated primary care in London over the past five years – the LIZ initiatives, a Primary-Care Led NHS, and the latest Primary Care Bill and White Papers. Their purposed has been to mould the publicly-owned health service into one which best meets the needs of the population within available resources.

We believe that if such objectives are to be achieved, London needs a primary care/GP workforce which has been appropriately educated from the point of entry into medical school and onwards throughout an individual's working life.

London has benefited recently from certain workforce and educational initiatives designed specifically to bring the elements of education and service closer together. In addition, the medical schools have begun the process of devolving the education of medical students into the primary care world and the undergraduate and postgraduate educational sectors have been working much more closely together.

In signing up to this statement we are confirming our belief that links between education and service should be further nurtured and developed, not only for GPs, but also for other stakeholders in primary care to ensure that London's patients receive primary care from high quality professionals.

Dr Steward Drage
Dr Neil Jackson
Professor Patrick Pietroni
Dr Tony Stanton
Professor Paul Wallace